D0927582

POST-STROKE REHABILITATION

CLINICAL PRACTICE GUIDELINE

Post-Stroke Rehabilitation Guideline Panel

Glen E. Gresham, MD (Chair)
Pamela W. Duncan, PhD, PT (Co-Chair)
William B. Stason, MD (Project Director)
Harold P. Adams, Jr., MD
Alan M. Adelman, MD, MS
David N. Alexander, MD
Duane S. Bishop, MD
Leonard Diller, PhD
Nancy E. Donaldson, RN, DNSc
Carl V. Granger, MD
Audrey L. Holland, PhD
Margaret Kelly-Hayes, EdD, RN, CRRN
Fletcher H. McDowell, MD
Larry Myers, MD
Marion A. Phipps, RN, MS, CRRN, FAAN
Elliot J. Roth, MD
Hilary C. Siebens, MD
Gloria A. Tarvin, MSW, LSW
Catherine Anne Trombly, ScD, OTR/L, FAOTA

U.S. Department of Health and Human Services
Public Health Service
Agency for Health Care Policy and Research
Rockville, Maryland

Formerly Published as AHCPR Publication No. 95-0662, May 1995

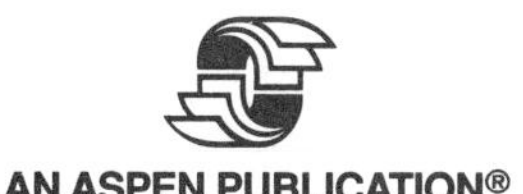

AN ASPEN PUBLICATION®
Aspen Publishers, Inc.
Gaithersburg, Maryland
1996

MOUNT CARMEL HEALTH
MOTHER CONSTANTINE LIBRARY
793 WEST STATE STREET
COLUMBUS, OH 43222

Library of Congress Cataloging-in-Publication Data

Post-Stroke Rehabilitation Guideline Panel.
Post-stroke rehabilitation : clinical practice guideline / Post-Stroke
Rehabilitation Guideline Panel : Glen E. Gresham … [et al.]
p. cm.
Originally published : Rockville, MD : U.S. Dept. of Health and Human
Services, Public Health Service, Agency for Health Care Policy and
Research, 1995. (Clinical practice guideline : no. 16) (AHCPR
publication : no. 95-0662)
Includes bibliographical references and index.
ISBN 0-8342-0811-3
1. Cerebrovascular disease--Patients--Rehabilitation--Standards.
I. Gresham, Glen E. II. Title.
[DNLM: 1. Cerebrovascular Disorders--rehabilitation.
2. Cerebrovascular Disorders--diagnosis. WL 355 U574p 1995a]
RC388.5.P63 1996
616.8' 1--dc20
DNLM/DLC
for Library of Congress
95-44619
CIP

Aspen Publishers, Inc.

Editorial Resources: Ruth Bloom

Library of Catalog Card Number: 95-44619
ISBN: 0-8342-0811-3

Printed in the United States of America

1 2 3 4 5

Foreword

This guideline was developed to assist primary care providers and rehabilitation specialists in the care of patients with disabilities from stroke and to help patients and their families become better informed consumers of rehabilitation services. The guideline seeks to increase awareness of the value and limitations of rehabilitation treatments after stroke and to encourage appropriate use of services.

Stroke is a leading cause of disability in the elderly and a significant cause of disability in younger people. Nearly 3 million Americans have some degree of disability from strokes, and the estimated annual economic burden is more than $30 billion. Rehabilitation attempts to reduce levels of disability and facilitate return to active and productive lives through a combination of educational, counseling, physical, and technology-based interventions. Prevention of recurrent strokes and prevention of complications from stroke are additional objectives. Rehabilitation combines a medical/scientific orientation with a social service orientation. Caring, support, and advocacy for the disabled are intrinsic components.

This guideline focuses primarily on the patient with a first stroke who has some degree of hemiparesis, with or without other neurological deficits, and is a candidate for treatment in an interdisciplinary rehabilitation program. Many recommendations also apply, however, to people with multiple strokes and those with limited disabilities who require care by a single rehabilitation discipline. Recommendations cover the period from the time of admission to an acute care hospital through any rehabilitation program and the transition to a community residence.

The benefits of rehabilitation must be distinguished from spontaneous neurological recovery after a stroke. For this reason, the natural history of recovery from stroke is emphasized. Recommendations address rehabilitation interventions during acute care, assessment strategies throughout acute care and rehabilitation, the choice of a rehabilitation setting, goal setting and management during rehabilitation, and issues that arise after the patient returns to a community residence. Recommendations are explicit where this is possible; otherwise, they imply a sense of priority or direction. Recommendations are supported by direct evidence from controlled trials where this is available. However, the sparsity of good scientific evidence has necessitated heavy reliance on expert opinion to support most recommendations.

The guideline was developed by the Center for Health Economics Research in Waltham, Massachusetts, under a contract with the Agency for Health Care Policy and Research (AHCPR). Development was led by a multidisciplinary panel of experts. Inputs included an extensive review of relevant literature, public testimony at a national public forum, and thorough review by a wide array of additional experts, professional

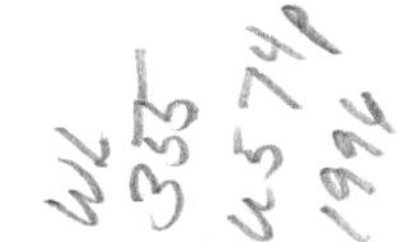

organizations, and rehabilitation facilities. These multiple levels of review substantially shaped the final document.

It is important to emphasize that this guideline is a first attempt to codify stroke rehabilitation practice. We hope it will provide useful guidance. Additional research is urgently needed to put stroke rehabilitation on a firm scientific footing. Results of this research need to be incorporated into revisions of the guideline.

Post-Stroke Rehabilitation Guideline Panel

Abstract

Stroke is a leading cause of disability in older persons and an important cause of disability in younger people. Rehabilitation aims to hasten and maximize recovery from stroke by treating the disabilities caused by the stroke. It serves to restore function, teach people with disabilities new ways to perform daily activities, and provide critical education and support for the stroke survivor and family.

This *Clinical Practice Guideline* is intended for the use of practitioners who are responsible for the patient's care during each phase of recovery, from the acute hospitalization through subsequent rehabilitation, and after return home or to another community residence.

Guideline recommendations focus on:

- The importance of thorough, consistent, and well-documented assessment at each stage of recovery to guide treatment decisions and monitor patient progress.
- Early implementation of rehabilitation interventions during acute care to facilitate recovery and prevent complications.
- Selection of the type of rehabilitation program or services best suited to the patient's needs.
- Establishment of realistic rehabilitation goals and provisions of treatment in accordance with a carefully developed rehabilitation management plan.
- The importance of combined followup and treatment during transition to a community residence.

Emphasis is given throughout to the importance of active patient and family involvement during all stages of recovery.

Recommendations depend heavily on expert opinion, since scientific evidence on the efficacy of rehabilitation programs or individual interventions is limited. Further research is urgently needed. Nonetheless, adherence to these guidelines should help to reduce the variations that currently exist in stroke rehabilitation practices and lead to more effective use of rehabilitation facilities.

Gresham GE, Duncan PW, Stason WB, et al. *Post-Stroke Rehabilitation.* Clinical Practice Guideline, No. 16. Rockville, MD: U.S. Department of Health and Human Services. Public Health Service, Agency for Health Care Policy and Research. AHCPR Publication No. 95-0662. May 1995.

The Agency for Health Care Policy and Research (AHCPR) was established in December 1989 under Public Law 101-239 (Omnibus Budget Reconciliation Act of 1989) to enhance the quality, appropriateness, and effectiveness of health care services and access to these services. AHCPR carries out its mission by conducting and supporting general health services research, including medical effectiveness research, facilitating development of clinical practice guidelines, and disseminating research findings and guidelines to health care providers, policymakers, and the public.

The legislation also established within AHCPR the Office of the Forum for Quality and Effectiveness in Health Care (the Forum). The Forum has primary responsibility for facilitating the development, periodic review, and updating of clinical practice guidelines. The guidelines will assist practitioners in the prevention, diagnosis, treatment, and management of clinical conditions.

Other AHCPR components include the following. The Center for Medical Effectiveness Research has principal responsibility for patient outcomes research and studies of variations in clinical practice. The Center for General Health Services Extramural Research supports research on primary care, the cost and financing of health care, and access to care for underserved and rural populations. The Center for General Health Services Intramural Research uses large data sets for policy research on national health care expenditures and utilization, hospital studies, and long-term care. The Center for Research Dissemination and Liaison produces and disseminates findings from AHCPR-supported research, including guidelines, and conducts research on dissemination methods. The Office of Health Technology Assessment responds to requests from Federal health programs for assessment of health care technologies. The Office of Science and Data Development develops specialized data bases and enhances techniques for using existing data bases for patient outcomes research.

Guidelines are available in formats suitable for health care practitioners, the scientific community, educators, and consumers. AHCPR invites comments and suggestions from users for consideration in development and updating of future guidelines. Please send written comments to Director, Office of the Forum for Quality and Effectiveness in Health Care, AHCPR, Willco Building, Suite 310, 6000 Executive Boulevard, Rockville, MD 20852.

Panel Members

Glen E. Gresham, MD, *Chair*
Professor and Chairman
Department of
Rehabilitation Medicine
State University of New York
at Buffalo
Director of
Rehabilitation Medicine
Erie County Medical Center
Buffalo, NY
Specialty: Internal Medicine

Pamela W. Duncan, PhD, PT, *Co-Chair*
Associate Professor,
Health Services Administration
University of Kansas
Director of Research,
Center on Aging
Kansas University Medical Center
Kansas City, KS
Specialty: Physical Therapy; Epidemiology; Health Services

Harold P. Adams, Jr., MD
Professor of Neurology
Director, Division of
Cerebrovascular Diseases
University of Iowa
College of Medicine
Iowa City, IA
Specialty: Neurology

Alan M. Adelman, MD, MS
Associate Professor and
Director of Research
Department of Family and
Community Medicine
Pennsylvania State University
The Milton S. Hershey
Medical Center
Hershey, PA
Specialty: Family Practice

David N. Alexander, MD
Director of Stroke Rehabilitation
Center for Diagnostic and
Rehabilitation Medicine
Daniel Freeman Hospital
Assistant Clinical Professor
Department of Neurology
University of California at
Los Angeles School of Medicine
Los Angeles, CA
Specialty: Neurology

Duane S. Bishop, MD
Director, Rehabilitation Psychiatry
Rhode Island Hospital
Associate Professor
Department of Psychiatry
Brown University
Providence, RI
Specialty: Psychiatry

Leonard Diller, PhD
Chief, Behavioral Science
Professor, Clinical Rehabilitation
Medicine
Rusk Institute of
Rehabilitation Medicine
NYU Medical Center
New York, NY
Specialty: Psychology

Nancy E. Donaldson, RN, DNSc
Consumer Representative
Newport Beach, CA
Specialty: Spousal/Family Caregiving—Consumer Perspective

Carl V. Granger, MD
Professor of
Rehabilitation Medicine
Director, Center for
Functional Assessment Research
State University of New York
at Buffalo
Buffalo, NY
Specialty: Physiatry

Audrey L. Holland, PhD
Professor and Head
Department of Speech
and Hearing Sciences
University of Arizona
Tucson, AZ
Specialty: Speech and Hearing Sciences; Speech-Language Pathology

Margaret Kelly-Hayes, EdD, RN, CRRN
Research Coordinator
and Investigator
Neuroepidemiology Section
Department of Neurology
Associate Clinical Professor
of Neurology
(Neurological Nursing)
Boston University
School of Medicine
Boston, MA
Specialty: Rehabilitation Nursing and Epidemiology

Fletcher H. McDowell, MD
Executive Medical Director
Burke Rehabilitation Hospital
White Plains, NY
Associate Dean
and Winifred Masterson Burke
Professor of Neurology
and Rehabilitation Medicine
Cornell University
Medical College
New York, NY
Specialty: Neurology

Larry R. Myers, MD
Family Practitioner Clinician
Ambulatory Sentinel
Practice Network
Community Preceptor
Mansfield, TX
Specialty: Family Practice

Marion A. Phipps, RN, MS, CRRN, FAAN
Rehabilitation Nurse Specialist
Beth Israel Hospital
Boston, MA
Specialty: Rehabilitation Nursing

Elliot J. Roth, MD
Medical Director
Rehabilitation Institute of Chicago
Professor, Department of Physical
Medicine and Rehabilitation
Northwestern University
Medical School
Chicago, IL
Specialty: Physiatry

Hilary C. Siebens, MD
Medical Director, Skilled Nursing
and Assessment Center
Medical Director,
Rehabilitation Research
Cedars-Sinai Medical Center
Assistant Clinical Professor
Department of Medicine,
Division of Physical Medicine
and Rehabilitation
University of California
at Los Angeles
Los Angeles, CA
Specialty: Geriatrics Physiatry

Gloria A. Tarvin, MSW, LSW
Chairperson of Allied Health/Nursing
Director of Social Work
Rehabilitation Institute of Chicago
Chicago, IL
Specialty: Social Work

Catherine Anne Trombly, ScD, OTR/L, FAOTA
Professor of Occupational Therapy
Sargent College of Allied Health Professions
Boston University
Boston, MA
Specialty: Occupational Therapy

Guideline Development and Use

Guidelines are systematically developed statements to assist practitioner and patient decisions about appropriate health care for specific clinical conditions. This guideline was written by an independent multidisciplinary panel of private-sector clinicians and other experts convened by the Agency for Health Care Policy and Research (AHCPR). The panel employed explicit, science-based methods and expert clinical judgment to develop specific statements on patient assessment and management for the clinical condition selected.

Extensive literature searches were conducted and critical reviews and syntheses were used to evaluate empirical evidence and significant outcomes. Peer review and field review were undertaken to evaluate the validity, reliability, and utility of the guideline in clinical practice. The panel's recommendations are primarily based on the published scientific literature. When the scientific literature was incomplete or inconsistent in a particular area, the recommendations reflect the professional judgment of panel members and consultants.

The guideline reflects the state of knowledge, current at the time of publication, on effective and appropriate care. Given the inevitable changes in the state of scientific information and technology, periodic review, updating, and revision will be done.

We believe that the AHCPR-assisted clinical guidelines will make positive contributions to the quality of care in the United States. We encourage practitioners and patients to use the information provided in this *Clinical Practice Guideline*. The recommendations may not be appropriate for use in all circumstances. Decisions to adopt any particular recommendation must be made by the practitioner in light of available resources and circumstances presented by individual patients.

Clifton R. Gaus, ScD
Administrator
Agency for Health Care Policy and Research

Publication of this guideline does not necessarily represent endorsement by the U.S. Department of Health and Human Services.

Acknowledgments

The panel and project director wish to give special thanks to the individuals, professional groups, and members of the rehabilitation facilities that contributed their time and expertise to the development of this guideline.

Several consultants to the panel helped immeasurably in identifying key issues, compiling relevant literature, and critiquing manuscript drafts of the guideline. These persons were Robert Berrian, MA, CTRS, Director of Recreational Therapy Services, Health South Rehabilitation Center, Pennsylvania; Richard W. Bohannon, EdD, PT, NCS, University of Connecticut; James S. Liljestrand, MD, MPH, Medical Director, Braintree Hospital, Massachusetts; and, Fay W. Whitney, RN, PhD, FAAN, School of Nursing, University of Pennsylvania.

Thomas Chalmers, MD, and Sidney Klawansky, MD, PhD, both from the Harvard School of Public Health, conducted the initial literature searches and performed meta-analyses on the benefits of stroke units, biofeedback, and functional electrical stimulation. These studies provided useful insights that facilitated interpretation of the scientific literature.

Expert peer reviewers of an early manuscript version of the guideline provided invaluable assistance in refining recommendations and marshalling additional supporting evidence from the scientific literature. The comprehensiveness of these reviews was outstanding. Professional organizations that reviewed the guideline documents, and practitioners and rehabilitation facilities who performed pilot testing, offered many constructive comments that we hope and expect will facilitate acceptance of the guideline's recommendations.

Ann Venable's expert editorial skills were essential to creating the AHCPR-sponsored *Clinical Practice Guideline* and *Quick Reference Guide for Clinicians* from a much longer *Guideline Technical Report*, and to writing the *Patient and Family Guide* (consumer version). We also wish to thank A. James Lee, PhD, for managing the project at the Center for Health Economics Research (Massachusetts), and Cheryl S. Lewis; Carol Ammering; Monika Reti; Holly Cyr; Joyce Huber, PhD; Helen Margulis; Robyn Tarantino; Philip W. Tyo; Adam Falk; and Amy Rensko for their able technical assistance.

We would like to thank David C. Lanier, MD, for his guidance and encouragement throughout the guideline's developmental process. He served as the project officer from the Office of the Forum for Quality and Effectiveness in Health Care, AHCPR. We are also grateful to Timothy F. Campbell of AHCPR for serving as managing editor of the guideline documents, and to Valna Montgomery for serving as AHCPR's product manager.

Contents

Tables

Figures

Attachments

Executive Summary

Introduction

Stroke is the third leading cause of death in the United States and the leading cause of disability among adults. Approximately 550,000 people suffer strokes each year and nearly 150,000 people die from them, while 3 million people are alive following strokes with varying degrees of neurological impairment. Consequent burdens in human and economic terms are enormous.

Brain infarctions account for about three-quarters of strokes and intracerebral or subarachnoid hemorrhages for about 15 percent; the remainder are of other or unknown causes. Stroke frequency increases dramatically with increasing age, doubling with every decade after 55 years of age. Men experience strokes more frequently than women and African Americans more frequently than whites. Mortality from stroke in different reports ranges from 17 to 34 percent in the first 30 days and from 25 to 40 percent in the first year. Stroke mortality has declined in recent years due to a combination of better acute care, reduced stroke severity, and earlier and more accurate diagnosis. Important modifiable risk factors include hypertension, cigarette smoking, atrial fibrillation, left ventricular hypertrophy, and transient ischemic attacks.

Hemiparesis is a presenting finding in three-quarters of patients. Acute neurological impairments frequently resolve spontaneously, but persisting disabilities lead to partial or total dependence in activities of daily living in 25 to 50 percent of stroke survivors.

Disablement has been conceptualized by the World Health Organization in terms of impairment (organ dysfunction), disability (difficulty with tasks), and handicap (social disadvantage). Rehabilitation is a restorative and learning process which seeks to hasten and maximize recovery from stroke by treating the resultant impairments, disabilities, and handicaps. It attempts to help the patient regain freedom of movement and functional independence and to reintegrate as fully as possible into community life.

The goal of this guideline is to improve the effectiveness of stroke rehabilitation by identifying the most effective methods of assessing and treating people who have disabilities due to stroke. The primary focus is on the patient with a first stroke who has developed hemiparesis with or without other neurological impairments. Recommendations refer to each stage of recovery, from the acute hospitalization through subsequent rehabilitation and return to a community residence. Target audiences for the guideline are practitioners who care for the stroke survivor during this period, and include both primary care physicians and rehabilitation professionals.

Scientific data supporting the effectiveness of rehabilitation programs and interventions in improving patient outcomes are limited. Wherever available, these data are used to support recommendations; where they are not available, reliance is placed on expert opinion. The need for post-stroke rehabilitation practice guidelines is underscored by the magnitude of the problem of disability from stroke, and also by wide variations in rehabilitation practices in the United States. Practice guidelines can help to reduce practice variations while, at the same time, encouraging better documentation of the benefits of rehabilitation services and implementation of the research that is needed to put stroke rehabilitation on a firm scientific footing.

Recommendations for Patient Management

Basic Principles of Rehabilitation

Interdisciplinary Care. Stroke rehabilitation frequently involves the services of several rehabilitation disciplines. The skills required depend on the nature of the patient's neurological deficits. Medical specialties that are commonly involved include physical medicine and rehabilitation (physiatry), neurology, geriatrics, internal medicine, psychiatry, and family practice. Consulting physicians from other specialties are called on as needed. Therapists include persons specializing in occupational therapy, physical therapy, psychology and neuropsychology, recreational therapy, and speech-language pathology. Other professionals who commonly participate include rehabilitation nurses, physician assistants, social workers, and dietitians. In many programs, physicians and rehabilitation clinicians work together as an interdisciplinary team.

Patient Assessment. Thorough, consistent, and fully documented assessment is required throughout the rehabilitation process. Assessment needs to include both repeated clinical examinations and the use of standardized instruments. Primary targets of assessment are neurological deficits; medical problems; physical, cognitive, emotional, and speech and language disabilities; and impediments to community reintegration. In the latter respect, assessment of the living environment, family functioning, and community supports is important. Assessment measures need to be valid, sensitive, and reliable if they are to measure progress accurately. This guideline recommends assessment protocols for each phase of rehabilitation and includes only the better validated measurement instruments.

Continuity of Care. The typical stroke survivor receives care in multiple settings during the course of recovery. Care that begins in the acute hospital is continued in inpatient (hospital or nursing facility), home, or outpatient rehabilitation programs, or by the family and the patient's personal physician or other health care provider after discharge. Since any change in treatment setting is accompanied by an increased risk of gaps in care, close communication among providers and between providers and the patient and family is essential. Thorough documentation and transfer of clinical information are especially important.

Patient and Family Involvement. Stroke survivors and, when relevant, families need to be fully informed and intimately involved in all rehabilitation decisions—the selection of rehabilitation setting, determination of rehabilitation goals and interventions, and choice of community residence. Rehabilitation is a learning experience in which both the patient and family are active participants. Ample opportunity needs to be given to address questions and concerns and to ensure adequate preparation during each stage of recovery.

Rehabilitation During the Acute Hospitalization

Stroke rehabilitation should begin as soon as the diagnosis of stroke is established and life-threatening problems are under control. Highest priorities are to prevent complications from the present stroke, prevent recurrent stroke, and mobilize the patient and encourage resumption of self-care activities as soon as medically feasible.

A considerable body of evidence, mainly from countries in Western Europe, indicates that better clinical outcomes are achieved when patients with acute stroke are treated in a setting that provides coordinated, multidisciplinary stroke-related evaluation and services. Skilled staff, better organization of services, and earlier implementation of rehabilitation interventions appear to be important components.

The value of early mobilization has been amply demonstrated. Measures should begin with range-of-motion exercises and physiologically sound changes of position in bed on the day of admission, and should be followed by progressively increased levels of activity as soon as medically tolerated. Early mobilization also includes encouragement to resume self-care activities and socialization.

Etiologic-specific measures to prevent recurrent stroke should be implemented in all patients. Evidence of effectiveness is especially strong for carotid endarterectomy in patients with 70 to 99 percent obstruction of the carotid artery, use of anticoagulants in patients with nonvalvular atrial fibrillation or other cause of cardiac embolic stroke, and use of antiplatelet agents in patients who have had a transient ischemic attack (TIA).

The value of low-molecular-weight (LMW) heparin or low-dose heparin (LDH) to prevent deep vein thrombosis in immobilized patients with stroke is well supported. Warfarin, intermittent pneumatic compression, and elastic stockings are also effective. Appropriate measures should be implemented in all immobilized patients.

Swallowing problems (dysphagia) are common after stroke and may cause aspiration. The patient's ability to swallow should be assessed before oral intake is begun, and techniques to facilitate swallowing should be implemented in affected patients. A feeding gastrostomy or nasogastric tube may be required if the patient does not regain the ability to swallow safely.

Patients who have had seizures after stroke should be given anticonvulsant medication to prevent recurrent seizures. Maintenance of skin integrity, fall prevention, and management of bowel and bladder function are important. Indwelling urinary catheters should be used only with patients who cannot be otherwise managed and should be removed as soon as possible to avoid urinary tract infections or other complications.

Patient and family support and education are intrinsic components of acute care for stroke. Adequate understanding of the cause and manifestations of the stroke, its treatment, and the prognosis are particularly important, as is counseling to help the patient and family deal with their concerns. Discharge planning extends support and education, identifies a postdischarge setting, and seeks to ensure continuity of care.

Screening for Rehabilitation and Choice of a Setting

All stroke survivors need caring, support, and education, but only some need formal rehabilitation. People who recover completely from their strokes will not need rehabilitation, and others will be too incapacitated to benefit from rehabilitation. Between these extremes are people with varying degrees of disability. For these individuals, the goal should be to identify the best possible match between their needs and the capabilities of available rehabilitation facilities.

A screening examination for rehabilitation should be performed as soon as the patient's medical and neurological condition permit by a person who is experienced in rehabilitation and has no direct financial interest in the referral decision. The screening examination uses information recorded in the medical record, but also needs to include direct examination of the patient and use of a well-standardized disability (e.g., activities of daily living) instrument and mental status screening test.

Threshold criteria for admission to a comprehensive rehabilitation program are medical stability, the presence of a functional deficit, the ability to learn, and enough physical endurance to sit supported for at least 1 hour and to participate actively in rehabilitation to at least some extent. Admission to an interdisciplinary program should be limited to patients who have more than one type of disability and who therefore need the services of two or more rehabilitation disciplines; patients with a single disability can benefit from individual services, but do not need an interdisciplinary program.

Stroke rehabilitation can be conducted in inpatient rehabilitation hospitals or rehabilitation units in acute care hospitals, in nursing facilities with rehabilitation programs, in outpatient facilities, or in the home. Hospital programs are usually the most comprehensive and intense and have the best medical coverage. A few nursing facility programs are similar to hospital programs, but many are less comprehensive. The wide variability in the capabilities of nursing facility programs makes it incumbent on the referring physician or hospital to evaluate the capabilities of the program with specific reference to each patient's needs. Outpatient and home rehabilitation programs also vary widely in their comprehensiveness and intensity.

Patients who are medically unstable are not suitable for any rehabilitation program. Those who have complex medical problems that require frequent attention are usually better treated in facilities that have round-the-clock coverage not only by rehabilitation nurses and physicians, but also immediately available consultant services by other medical specialists. Patients with moderate or severe disabilities and sufficient physical endurance to tolerate intense rehabilitation (at least 3 hours of physically demanding exercises per day) are candidates for intense hospital or nursing facility programs. Patients with milder degrees of disability and those who have poor physical endurance or limited attention spans are usually better served by lower intensity programs in nursing facilities, at home, or in outpatient facilities. The characteristics of the home environment and availability of social support may affect the feasibility of home or outpatient rehabilitation; for the latter, availability of transportation can also be a constraint. In some instances, a further period of recuperation in a nursing facility or at home will allow enough recovery for a patient to enter a comprehensive rehabilitation program at a later time. Providers need to remain alert to these opportunities, and patients and families should be made aware that reassessment could occur in the future, leading to a change in treatment.

Managing Rehabilitation

Assessment. A summary of the patient's previous medical record and information collected during the screening examination should be available at the time of admission to any rehabilitation program, so that changes in the patient's condition can be identified and questions about medical management can be resolved promptly.

A thorough baseline rehabilitation evaluation should be completed within 3 working days of admission to an intense rehabilitation program (hospital or nursing facility), within 7 days of admission to a lower intensity nursing facility program, and within three visits in the case of an outpatient or home rehabilitation program. The initial history and physical examination by a physician and a nurse should be done within 24 hours or during the first visit. These timelines, reflecting expert opinion, attempt to establish a reasonable balance between feasibility and the need for prompt treatment.

Setting Rehabilitation Goals and Developing the Rehabilitation Management Plan. Rehabilitation goals should be realistic in terms of current levels of disability and potential for recovery, and should be mutually agreed to by the patient, family, and rehabilitation professionals.

It is important that goals be recorded in the medical record in explicit, measurable terms so that they can serve as yardsticks against which to measure the patient's progress during rehabilitation. The rehabilitation management plan specifies measures to prevent recurrent stroke and complications; treatments for comorbidities; and rehabilitation interventions with their sequence, intensity, frequency, and expected duration.

Monitoring Progress. The patient's progress should be monitored regularly during rehabilitation—weekly during intense inpatient rehabilitation in a hospital or nursing facility and at least every other week during less intense nursing facility, home, or outpatient programs. Clinical examinations and standardized instruments that focus on impairments or disabilities being treated should be used. The information obtained is valuable in measuring progress toward goals, identifying the need for changes to treatment regimens, and, ultimately, guiding discharge decisions.

Managing Functional Health Patterns. Management of dysphagia; maintenance of nutrition, hydration, and skin integrity; and management of bowel and bladder function remain as important as they were during acute care. Sleep disturbances are common and should receive cause-specific treatment.

Managing Sensorimotor Deficits. Patients with motor deficits but some motor control should be encouraged to move the affected limb in functional tasks and offered exercises and training directed at improving strength and motor control and improving performance. Available research evidence does not, however, support any superiority of neuromuscular facilitation over traditional physical therapy exercises, nor does it adequately support the value of biofeedback or functional electrical stimulation in enhancing responses to physical therapy.

Compensatory Training. Patients with persistent functional deficits should be taught new approaches to performing important tasks of daily living, using the affected limb when possible or, when not, the unaffected limb. This recommendation is supported primarily by expert opinion and applies to the performance of a wide range of tasks including self-care (ADL) tasks; more complex tasks required during independent living such as the use of the telephone and public transportation, driving a car, and financial management; and performance of social and recreational activities, spiritual roles, and work. Adaptive devices should be used if other methods to perform the task are not available or cannot be learned, and to facilitate task performance if easy fatigability or patient safety are factors.

Managing Cognitive and Perceptual Deficits. Cognitive and perceptual deficits increase the severity of functional deficits, affect rehabilitation goals, and require highly goal-directed rehabilitation plans.

Diagnosing and Treating Depression. Depression is common after stroke. Diagnosis requires a high level of suspicion and a thorough clinical examination by a mental health professional. Depression scales are useful for screening and for monitoring responses to treatment, but should not be relied on for diagnosis. The choice of treatment depends on the cause of depression, the severity of symptoms, and responses to treatment. Drug treatment, psychotherapy, or a combination may be needed in patients with major depression; mild depression often responds to counseling and encouragement. Initial doses of drugs should be small, and the patient should be closely monitored for side effects.

Managing Speech and Language Disorders. Problems in functional communication are common after stroke. Thorough evaluation requires the use of standardized evaluation measures. A variety of approaches to treatment have been used in patients with aphasia and appear to be effective in some patients. However, treatments of right hemisphere communication disorders, dysarthria, and apraxia of speech have been less extensively studied.

Discharge Planning. Discharge planning should begin on the day of admission. It should be coordinated by one person, but should involve the stroke survivor, family/caregivers, and relevant rehabilitation professionals. Goals are to identify a safe place of residence, ensure adequate patient and family education, and arrange for continued medical care, rehabilitation, and community services. Decisions ideally reflect a consensus of all involved parties.

Discharge from an inpatient rehabilitation program should be considered when rehabilitation goals have been achieved or when 2 weeks have elapsed without documented progress. Under these circumstances, transfer to another level of care or discharge is usually in the patient's best interests and also represents a cost-effective use of rehabilitation resources. Exceptions occur when there is a clear explanation for a temporary functional plateau.

Assessments prior to discharge include evaluation of the patient's functional status, adequacy of the proposed living environment, adequacy of support by family or other caregivers, and availability of community supports.

Transition to the Community

Return to a community residence after an acute hospitalization for stroke, or after an inpatient rehabilitation program, can be difficult for the stroke survivor and family alike. At this time, the person has to assume increased responsibility for independent functioning in the absence of the supportive environment of the inpatient setting, with the family or other caregivers providing needed support. Continuity of services is important during this period, and patient and family counseling may be needed to facilitate family functioning and improve outcomes.

The patient's continuing needs for medical care and rehabilitation should be coordinated by a single clinician in collaboration with the individual and family. An initial visit with this care coordinator should be scheduled no later than 1 month after discharge. Close communication among providers, the patient, and the family is critical to developing a coherent care plan and avoiding gaps or inconsistencies in care.

After the return to a community residence, progress needs to be evaluated at regular intervals to document whether the person is maintaining gains made during rehabilitation, progressing toward more independent function, and successfully reintegrating with the family and community.

Rehabilitation services generally should be phased out slowly after completion of hospital or nursing facility rehabilitation programs or during home or outpatient programs to avoid the feeling of abandonment and provide opportunities for "tuneups." Continued rehabilitation services should be justified, however, by documented evidence of progress.

Community supports are important for many stroke survivors. Acute care hospitals and rehabilitation facilities should maintain up-to-date information on community resources and offer assistance to patients and their families in obtaining needed services. Individual health care providers should be familiar with available services and sources of information.

Issues that arise after return to a community residence include safety and fall prevention, health promotion, sexuality, resumption of leisure and community activities, driving, and return to work. Each of these areas needs to be carefully addressed.

Research Priorities

Research is needed to fill gaps in knowledge regarding the effectiveness of stroke rehabilitation. Highest priority should be given to well-controlled experimental studies that assess functional and quality-of-life outcomes and the cost effectiveness of alternative service delivery strategies.

Goals should be to:

- Identify the characteristics of patients who are most likely to benefit from rehabilitation interventions.
- Determine the optimal type of rehabilitation program for different types of patients.
- Identify factors that affect the optimal timing, intensity, and duration of rehabilitation.
- Determine the effectiveness of specific treatments or combinations of treatments in reducing impairments and improving function.
- Develop and validate standardized tests for use in monitoring post-stroke rehabilitation.

1 Overview

Goals of the Guideline

The primary goal of this guideline is to improve the effectiveness of rehabilitation in helping the person with disabilities from a stroke to achieve the best possible functional outcome and quality of life. The central focus is on the patient with a first stroke (of any etiology) who has developed hemiparesis with or without other neurological impairments and is a candidate for treatment in an interdisciplinary rehabilitation program. Most recommendations also apply to people with other neurological impairments from stroke, those with recurrent strokes, and those who may need limited rehabilitation services but not a comprehensive program. The emphasis is on what is best for the patient and the patient's family. Provider and reimbursement issues, while important, are not addressed in detail. Specific goals are to:

- Make available to rehabilitation professionals and primary care providers the best current knowledge and expert consensus regarding effective rehabilitation practices.
- Improve the public's and medical community's understanding of stroke rehabilitation services and their strengths and limitations.
- Improve access to rehabilitation services by increasing the awareness of patients, families, health professionals, and the public at large of the availability and capabilities of these services.
- Emphasize the patient- and family-centered nature of rehabilitation and the importance of capitalizing on patient, family, and community strengths and potentials during the rehabilitation process.
- Enhance community integration of the stroke survivor with disabilities.
- Encourage rehabilitation professionals to reexamine their practice patterns, and to target services at patients who are most likely to benefit.
- Stimulate future research to fill critical gaps in our knowledge regarding the effectiveness of stroke rehabilitation.

What Is Stroke Rehabilitation?

An established and universally accepted definition for stroke is "acute neurologic dysfunction of vascular origin . . . with symptoms and signs corresponding to the involvement of focal areas of the brain" (World Health Organization, 1989). It can also be described as the rapid onset of neurological deficits that persist for at least 24 hours and are caused either by intracerebral or subarachnoid hemorrhage or by partial or complete blockage of a blood vessel supplying or draining a part of the brain, leading to the infarction of brain tissue. A stroke is distinguished from a transient ischemic attack (TIA) by the fact that neurological deficits in TIAs clear spontaneously within 24 hours.

Stroke rehabilitation is a restorative learning process which seeks to hasten and maximize recovery from stroke by treating the disabilities caused by the stroke, and to prepare the stroke survivor to reintegrate as fully as possible into community life. Approaches to rehabilitation include:

- Prevention of secondary complications.
- Remediation, or treatment to reduce neurological deficits.
- Compensation to offset and adapt to residual disabilities.
- Maintenance of function over the long term.

Operationally, rehabilitation encompasses a broad array of biomedical, social, educational, and vocational interventions that can be provided in a variety of institutional and community settings. Rehabilitation professionals include physiatrists, neurologists with special interests in rehabilitation, internists, family physicians, geriatricians, rehabilitation nurses, physician assistants, physical therapists, occupational therapists, speech-language pathologists, psychologists, psychiatrists, social workers, vocational rehabilitation specialists, recreational therapists, orthotists, and dietitians. Services are often provided by an interdisciplinary team in which the specific participants will depend on the patient's physical, cognitive, and emotional disabilities and the availability of rehabilitation resources in the community.

Need for a Guideline

The need for a stroke rehabilitation guideline stems from the magnitude of the human and economic burdens that result from stroke; wide variations in practice patterns among different communities and treatment settings; and continued controversy over the benefits of stroke rehabilitation.

Stroke is the third leading cause of death in the United States and is the leading cause of long-term disability among adults. Approximately 550,000 people suffer a stroke each year, nearly 150,000 people die from stroke, and about 3 million stroke survivors have varying degrees of residual neurological impairment (American Heart Association, 1991; Prescott, 1994). Stroke incidence doubles with each successive decade over 55 years of age (Dyken, Wolf, Barnett, et al., 1984). Incidence is about 30 percent higher in men than in women (Wolf, Cobb, and D'Agostino, 1992), about 50 percent higher in African-American men than in white men, and 2.3 times higher in African-American women than in white women (Gillum, 1988). The economic burden from stroke has been estimated to be $30 billion in health care costs and lost productivity each year (Matchar, McCrory, Barnett, et al., 1994).

Rehabilitation practice patterns in the United States vary greatly from one geographic area to another, reflecting an uneven distribution of rehabilitation facilities and professionals, differing thresholds for admission to inpatient facilities, and differences in treatment regimens. An analysis of Medicare claims for rehabilitation services received in 1991, commissioned by the Agency for Health Care Policy and Research as part of this guideline development process, found that 17 percent of patients who survived their strokes were admitted to a hospital-based inpatient rehabilitation program, 23 percent were treated in a nursing facility, and 40 percent received outpatient or home care rehabilitation services. A total of 73 percent received services in one or more of these types of settings.

These wide practice variations occurred in the face of limited evidence supporting the effectiveness of stroke rehabilitation. Though observational studies provide a wealth of information on the natural history and epidemiology of stroke, few well-controlled clinical studies document benefits from rehabilitation. Most clinical studies have focused on short-term changes in impairment or function during inpatient rehabilitation. Results have been inconsistent, and where they favor the experimental group, the difference is generally small. A particularly difficult problem has been that of distinguishing rehabilitation effects from spontaneous neurological recovery after a stroke. The most convincing evidence that rehabilitation may be effective is provided by studies that have examined the effects of treatment in stroke patients with chronic neurological impairments, thereby excluding effects of spontaneous recovery, which largely occurs during the first 6 months following a stroke.

Technical deficiencies that compromise the validity of many studies include suboptimal study designs, small sample sizes, highly selected study populations, failure to control for length of time since stroke onset, incompletely described interventions, unstandardized measures of outcome, and inadequate statistical methodologies (Dombovy, Sandok, and Basford, 1986; Ernst, 1990; Stineman and Granger, 1991).

The scarcity of scientific evidence supporting the benefits of rehabilitation has mixed implications for the guideline. On the one hand, it detracts from the strength of scientific support for recommendations and necessitates heavy reliance on professional judgment and expert opinion. On the other hand, the scarcity of evidence creates the opportunity to assess current knowledge, to develop guidelines that will help to move stroke rehabilitation toward consistent norms, and to stimulate the research that is needed to put individual interventions and comprehensive rehabilitation programs on firm scientific ground. This guideline is a first step and will need to be updated as new information becomes available.

Priorities for Future Research

Research is urgently needed to address critical questions about the effectiveness and cost effectiveness of stroke rehabilitation. Highest priority should be given to well-controlled experimental studies that assess functional performance and quality-of-life outcomes and the cost effectiveness of alternative service delivery strategies. Goals should be to:

- Identify the characteristics of patients who are most likely to benefit from rehabilitation.
- Determine the optimal program for rehabilitation for different types of patients.
- Identify factors that determine the optimal timing, intensity, and duration of rehabilitation.
- Determine the effectiveness of specific treatments or combinations of treatments in reducing impairments or improving function.
- Develop and validate standardized tests for use in monitoring post-stroke rehabilitation.

In most instances, preference should be given to single- or multiple-center randomized clinical trials because of their greater scientific validity. Ethical concerns about withholding treatment from stroke survivors can be overcome by using "usual care" rather than "no treatment" controls. Cohort and case-control studies can also yield valuable information if they are well designed and properly analyzed. Population-based studies that collect data prospectively on representative samples of patients with completed strokes are especially useful.

Framework for the Guideline

Conceptual Model

The goals of rehabilitation can be visualized according to the conceptual framework of disablement developed in the World Health Organization's (WHO) International Classification of Impairments, Disabilities, and Handicaps (ICIDH) (World Health Organization, 1980) and Nagi's "functional limitation" model (Nagi, 1965). The former classifies disablement in terms of "disease," "impairment," "disability," and "handicap," in which **disease** is the underlying diagnosis and pathologic process, **impairment** is the loss or abnormality of physical or psychological capacities, **disability** is a restriction or lack of ability of a person to perform an activity in daily life, and **handicap** is a disadvantage resulting from an impairment or disability that limits or prevents fulfillment of a role that is normal for that person.

Nagi, on the other hand, emphasizes "pathology," "impairment," "functional limitation," and "disability," where **pathology** is the "interruption or interference of normal bodily processes or structures"; **impairment** is "loss or abnormality of mental, emotional, physiological, or anatomical structure or function"; **functional limitation** is "restriction or lack of ability to perform an action or activity in the manner or within the range considered normal"; and **disability** is the "inability or limitation in performing socially defined activities and roles expected of individuals within a social or physical environment." The disability model envisioned by Nagi has the advantages of emphasizing the causative role of risk factors and the importance of the quality of life. "Disability" in Nagi's framework is equivalent to "handicap" in WHO's framework and avoids the negative implications attached to this term.

Figure 1 combines concepts from the Nagi and WHO models and relates them across three levels of concern: the organ level, person level, and societal level. At the organ level, pathology determines impairments. These contribute to disability or difficulty performing tasks at the person level. Disability, a central concept in this model, is also strongly influenced by contextual factors such as physical barriers, social and cultural factors, and the attitudes of those involved. Disability, in combination with societal expectations, contributes to handicap or social disadvantage at the societal level. The lower portion of Figure 1 shows how functional assessment and interventions differ for the three levels. Functional assessment determines unmet needs which then become the focus of medical or restorative, adaptive, environmental, or social interventions. This guideline adheres to the nomenclature shown in Figure 1, which is widely accepted by rehabilitation professionals.

Outcome Measures

Potential measures of the success of stroke rehabilitation include:

- Survival.
- Normalized health patterns (such as nutrition, continence, and sleep).
- Freedom from physical pain and emotional distress.
- Cognitive and communicative abilities.
- Freedom from impairments affecting motor control, mobility of joints, sensation, speech and language, and other areas.
- Independence in mobility and the basic activities of daily living.
- Independence in complex daily functions and social roles.
- Successful family function and adaptation.
- Quality of life.

Actual performance of a function is a better measure of success than the capacity to perform the function in the supportive environment of a rehabilitation program. Motivation, confidence, stimulation, and environmental factors can all strongly affect actual performance.

The ability of a person with a stroke to return home after treatment is usually regarded as a desirable outcome. This may not be the case, however, if the person's needs for physical care and support impose intolerable burdens on caregivers.

Scope of the Guideline

This guideline is intended for use by all of the professionals who participate in post-stroke rehabilitation. It is specifically directed at the patient with a first stroke who has residual hemiparesis with or without

Figure 1. Relationship of functional assessment and interventions to the World Health Organization's impairment, disability, and handicap model

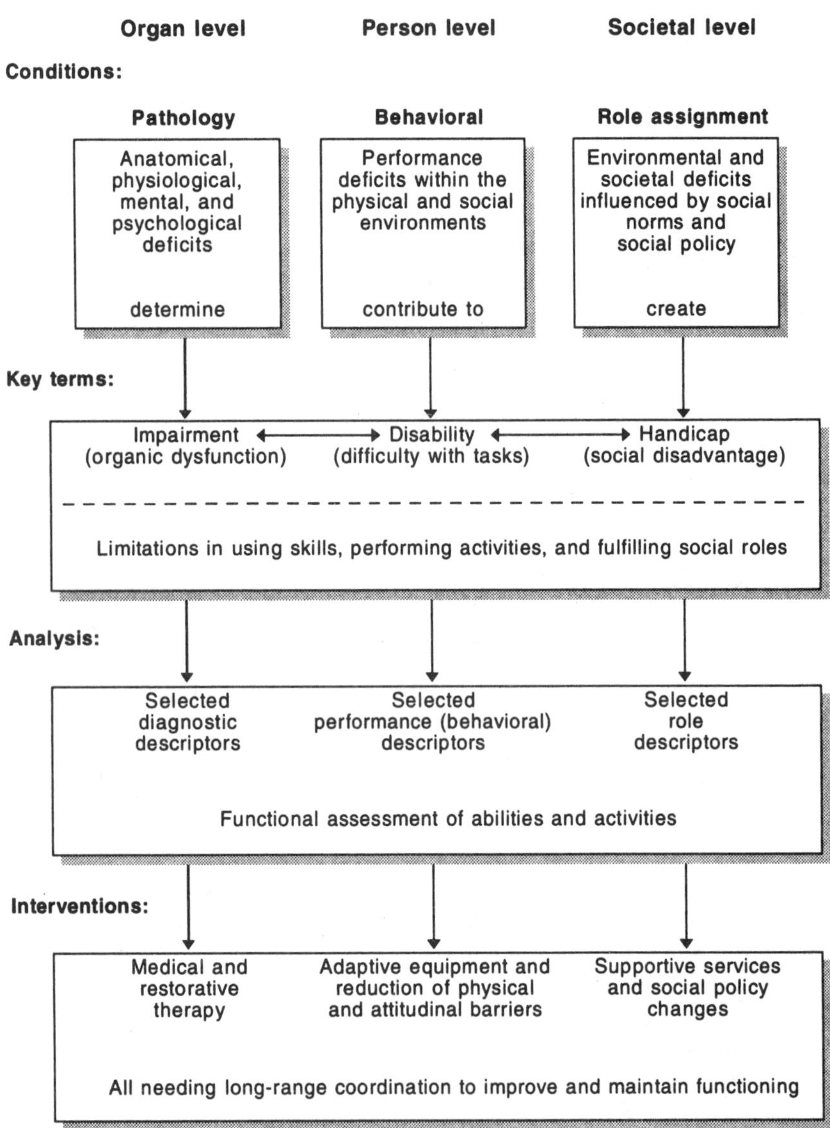

Source: Granger CV, Gresham GE, editors. Functional assessment in rehabilitation medicine. Baltimore, MD: Williams & Wilkins, 1984. p. 14–25. Used with permission.

other neurological impairments. Most recommendations will also apply to the person with a recurrent stroke or with stroke-related neurological impairments in the absence of hemiparesis.

The guideline addresses the rehabilitation needs of the person who has had a stroke from the acute hospital stay through subsequent rehabilitation and return to the community. Its scope corresponds to the clinical flow diagram for stroke rehabilitation shown in Figure 2. Most patients with strokes are initially admitted to a stroke unit or general medical service of an acute care hospital. The primary objectives of rehabilitation services are to prevent complications and to mobilize the patient, mentally as well as physically, as soon as medically feasible. Screening for rehabilitation is performed when the patient's condition has stabilized—often within 3 to 5 days if the clinical course is uncomplicated. Patients who recover completely will not need rehabilitation. Those who remain severely incapacitated are not likely to benefit at that time; however, they may improve sufficiently over a further period of recuperation and should be reevaluated at a later date.

Between these extremes are patients with persistent functional deficits who are potential candidates for individual rehabilitation services or an interdisciplinary program. The choice of rehabilitation setting will depend on careful evaluation of clinical findings and the capabilities of rehabilitation facilities in a given community. The fundamental components of any program are baseline assessment, development of rehabilitation goals and a plan for achieving them, implementation of interventions, and monitoring of progress.

When goals have been achieved or a plateau in progress has been reached, the patient is discharged from rehabilitation or transferred to another type of setting (e.g., to an outpatient or home program from an inpatient setting). Transition to a community residence or the cessation of rehabilitation services often raises difficult issues of adaptation and continuity of care that need to be addressed.

Nomenclature in Stroke Rehabilitation

This guideline employs a standard terminology to describe rehabilitation settings, programs, interventions, and participants. Following are definitions of some of the more important terms used. See the Glossary for other definitions.

Rehabilitation Settings. The terms used to describe various rehabilitation settings are:

- **Acute care hospital.** A full-service hospital where patients with an acute stroke are treated either in a medical service or in a specialized stroke unit, and where rehabilitation interventions are normally begun during the acute phase.
- **Inpatient rehabilitation.** Rehabilitation performed during an inpatient stay in a freestanding rehabilitation hospital or a rehabilitation unit of an

Figure 2. Clinical flow diagram for stroke rehabilitation

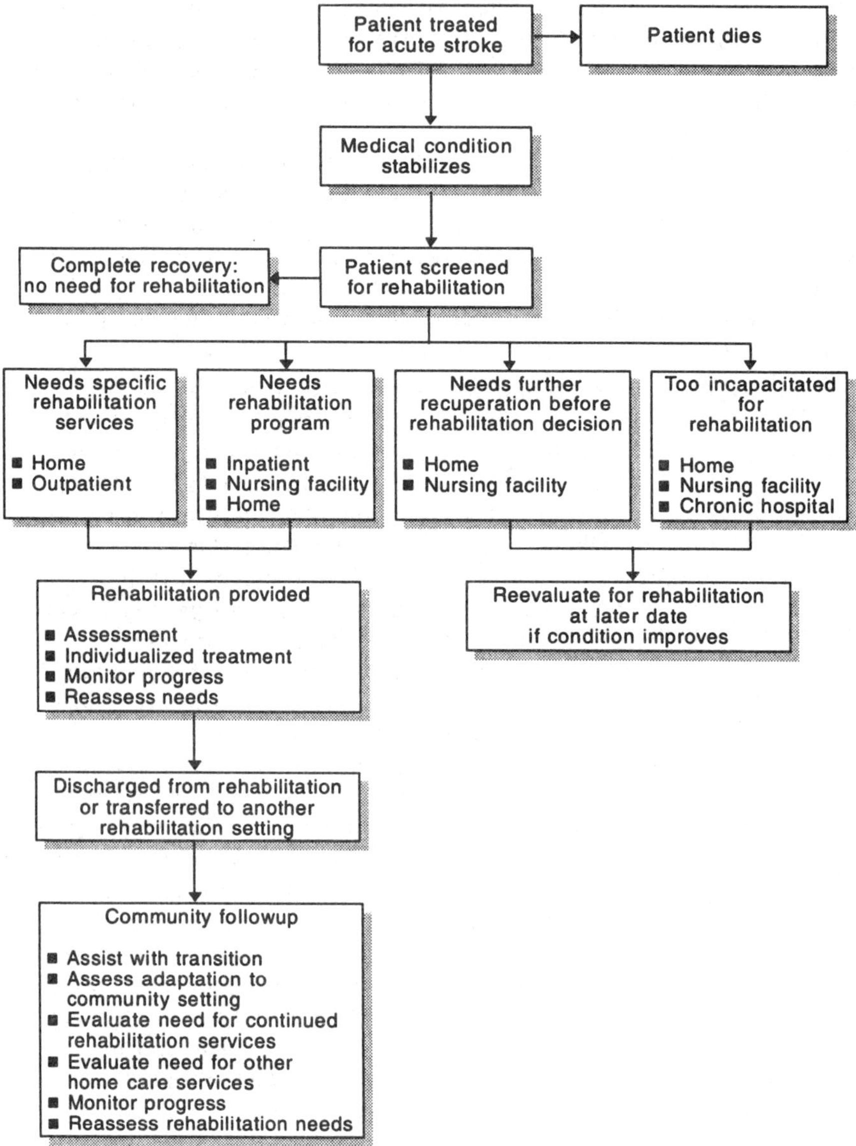

acute care hospital. The term **inpatient** is also used to refer generically to programs where the patient is in residence during treatment, whether in an acute care hospital, a rehabilitation hospital, or a nursing facility.

- **Nursing facility rehabilitation.** Rehabilitation performed during a stay in a nursing facility. Nursing facilities vary widely in their rehabilitation capabilities, ranging from maintenance care to comprehensive and intense rehabilitation programs.
- **Outpatient rehabilitation.** Rehabilitation performed in an outpatient facility that is either freestanding or attached to an acute care or rehabilitation hospital. Day hospital care is a subset of outpatient rehabilitation in which the patient spends a major part of the day in an outpatient rehabilitation facility.
- **Home-based rehabilitation.** A rehabilitation program provided in the patient's place of residence.

The Spectrum of Rehabilitation Care. Rehabilitation ranges from **individual services** by a single clinician or discipline for patients with circumscribed deficits to **comprehensive rehabilitation programs** that encompass multiple, interactive services provided by an interdisciplinary team. In between are **programs** of varying complexity which involve two or more rehabilitation disciplines, coordinated in some fashion.

Rehabilitation programs can also be described in terms of their intensity, measured as the number and duration of services per day or per week. In this guideline, an **intense** program involves two or more rehabilitation disciplines, 5 days a week, with a minimum of 3 hours of active rehabilitation each day. Less intense programs cover a wide range, from 1 hour of services two or three times a week upward.

Some sources use the term **acute rehabilitation** to denote inpatient hospital rehabilitation and **subacute rehabilitation** to denote a program conducted in a nursing facility. Instead, this guideline substitutes categories of intensity to describe the actual content of programs wherever they take place. The trend toward providing intense rehabilitation programs in nursing facilities and at home, as well as in hospitals, supports this approach.[1]

The Recipient of Rehabilitation Services. The guideline uses the term **patient** to refer to a recipient of a rehabilitation program or services regardless of setting. (In some sources, a distinction is made among settings, with a **patient** receiving services in an inpatient hospital rehabilitation program, a **resident** in a nursing facility, and a **client** in a

---

[1]The Commission on Accreditation of Rehabilitation Facilities (CARF) has proposed a new classification of accredited hospital and nursing facility programs into one "acute" and two "subacute" categories based on the intensity of rehabilitation provided and the medical and nursing needs of patients. The Joint Commission on Accreditation of Healthcare Organizations (JCAHO) is also considering distinguishing between "acute" and "subacute" levels of care.

home-based or outpatient program.) The term **stroke survivor** is often used in the guideline when referring to a person who has had a stroke but is not necessarily a patient at present (e.g., the person may have completed treatment and reentered the community) or when the focus of the discussion is on the person as an individual rather than as a patient. The terms **person** and **individual** are also used.

The Family and Caregivers. The term **family** is used broadly to include both relatives and friends with whom the patient was living before the stroke or who are close to the patient and involved in the patient's treatment. The term **caregiver** refers to the one or two individuals who provide most of the day-to-day support needed by the stroke survivor at home.

Methodology

Panel Selection and Guideline Development

Panel Selection. The guideline was developed by a panel of experts and consultants representing the medical and rehabilitation specialties involved in stroke rehabilitation. Medical specialties included family practice, geriatrics, internal medicine, neurology, physiatry, and psychiatry. Other rehabilitation specialties included occupational therapy, physical therapy, psychology, rehabilitation nursing, social work, speech-language pathology, and recreational therapy. Consumer representatives also helped with the development of the guideline. Each panelist was nominated by the relevant professional society and was approved by the Agency for Health Care Policy and Research.

Guideline Formulation. The steps in formulating the guideline were as follows:

- Establishment of the scope of the guideline, including clinical issues to be addressed, patient population to be emphasized, target audience, and the measures of patient benefits and harms by which the rehabilitation process or individual interventions should be evaluated.
- An extensive search of the scientific literature and literature on rehabilitation procedures, costs, practice variations, and other policy issues. Sources included MEDLINE, several social science data bases, published dissertations, and additional citations identified from the bibliographies of review articles and from recommendations by panel members or consultants. More than 1,900 articles were reviewed and are listed in the *Guideline Technical Report*, and nearly 500 are cited in this *Clinical Practice Guideline.* (See later description of these documents.) The primary emphasis has been on experimental studies, but review articles and observational studies have been included if they provided information critical to understanding the natural history of stroke or the effects of rehabilitation. Animal studies and manuscripts written in other than the English language were excluded.

- Analysis of Medicare claims for a nationwide 10-percent sample of beneficiaries with admission for stroke to an acute care hospital in 1991. This analysis obtained data on the utilization and costs of rehabilitation services received during the first 6 months following stroke and documented practice variations by geographic area.
- Extensive discussion of the evidence by the panel and related formulation of recommendations. Each recommendation was supported by at least 75 percent of panel members.
- Development of four documents: A comprehensive *Guideline Technical Report*, this *Clinical Practice Guideline* emphasizing guidance for practitioners, a *Quick Reference Guide for Clinicians*, and a *Patient and Family Guide.* The *Guideline Technical Report* includes an analysis of policy issues and recommendations for a research agenda in stroke rehabilitation.

External Review. Four stages of external review took place:

- An open forum in Washington, D.C., which provided an opportunity for professional and provider organizations, manufacturers, pharmaceutical firms, and individuals to present either written or oral statements. The 34 statements received provided valuable perspectives.
- Detailed review of the full *Guideline Technical Report* by 44 experts in disciplines involved in stroke rehabilitation. Reviewers were asked to identify errors of omission and interpretation and to review draft recommendations, reformulate them if appropriate, and justify the changes in terms of the scientific literature or professional experience. This review was extraordinarily helpful and resulted in significant changes in the guideline and its recommendations.
- Review of the *Clinical Practice Guideline*, the *Quick Reference Guide for Clinicians*, and the *Patient and Family Guide* by a broad array of professional, provider, insurer, and consumer organizations in order to obtain reactions to the guidelines, assess their potential effects on the practice and costs of stroke rehabilitation, and determine their sensitivity to patient, family, and clinician concerns. The review was especially important in obtaining the views of organizations that will be participants in guideline implementation.
- Pilot testing of the *Clinical Practice Guideline*, the *Quick Reference Guide for Clinicians*, and the *Patient and Family Guide* by 10 provider organizations that deliver rehabilitation services and one independent case-management consultant. Each respondent was asked to estimate the overall effects of the guideline on admission policies, procedures, and quality improvement activities and to test the guideline on patients who had received or were receiving rehabilitation services and record specific ways in which the guideline differed from current practice.

Format and Classification of Recommendations

Each guideline recommendation is justified in terms of the level of research evidence supporting it and the degree of consensus on it among panel members. The distinction between support derived from scientific studies and that derived from expert opinion is important. Well-performed and relevant scientific studies provide a higher standard of evidence when they are available, but many aspects of stroke rehabilitation have not been addressed by such studies. Expert judgments supplement research evidence by factoring in clinical experience and human values that are not easily captured in scientific studies, and by extrapolating from scientific findings that were obtained with specific populations under specific conditions to a broad clinical context.

Support for recommendations is characterized as follows:

Research Evidence:

A Supported by the results of two or more randomized controlled trials (RCTs) that have good internal validity, and also specifically address the question of interest in a group of patients comparable to the one to which the recommendation applies (external validity).

B Supported by a single RCT meeting the criteria given above for "A"-level evidence, by RCTs that only indirectly address the questions of interest, or by two or more nonrandomized clinical trials (case control or cohort studies) in which the experimental and control groups are demonstrably similar or multivariate analyses have effectively controlled for group differences.

C Supported by a single non-RCT meeting the criteria given above for "B"-level evidence, by studies using historical controls, or by studies using quasi-experimental designs such as pre- and post-treatment comparisons.

NA (not available). Recommendation is not addressed by experimental studies.

Expert Opinion:

Strong consensus. Agreement among 90 percent or more of panel members and expert reviewers.

Consensus. Agreement among 75 to 89 percent of panel members and expert reviewers.

Organization of the Guideline

Chapter 2 briefly describes the epidemiology and natural history of stroke, and Chapter 3 describes methods of assessment applicable to patients with strokes. Practice recommendations are presented in the next four chapters: Chapter 4 concerns rehabilitation during the acute phase of stroke treatment; Chapter 5, the screening for further rehabilitation and choice of a rehabilitation setting; Chapter 6, management of the rehabilitation process; and Chapter 7, discharge and the return to the community. The attachments provide information on the validity, reliability, and sensitivity of panel-preferred assessment instruments used with stroke patients.

2 Epidemiology and Natural History of Stroke

Epidemiology of Stroke

Information on stroke incidence and prevalence, mortality, etiology, and risk factors is summarized in Table 1.

Incidence and Prevalence

Stroke incidence, defined as the number of acute strokes per year, depends primarily on the age, sex, and race mix of the population, whether only first strokes or all strokes are counted, whether transient ischemic attacks (TIAs) are included as well as completed strokes, and the diagnostic criteria used.

The average age-adjusted incidence rate of first strokes has been reported to be 114 per 100,000 but ranges from 81 to 150 per 100,000 in different studies (Terent, 1993). Men have 30 to 80 percent higher rates than women (Broderick, Phillips, Whisnant, et al., 1989; Harmsen, Tsipogianni, and Wilhelmsen, 1992; Wolf, D'Agostino, O'Neal, et al., 1992). The incidence of stroke doubles with every decade after 55 years of age (Dyken, Wolf, Barnett, et al., 1984). In Rochester, Minnesota (1980 to 1984), incidence increased nearly ninefold between ages 55 to 64 and 85 years or over (Broderick, Phillips, Whisnant, et al., 1989). Stroke rates are 50 percent higher in African-American men than in white men, and 130 percent higher in African-American women than in white women (Gillum, 1988).

First-ever strokes account for about 75 percent of acute events and recurrent strokes for about 25 percent (Terent, 1993). The recurrence rate is 7 to 10 percent per year and is highest in the first year after a first stroke. In the Framingham Study, recurrence was found to be particularly common for thrombotic stroke and more frequent in men (Sacco, Wolf, Kannel, et al., 1982).

Stroke prevalence—the number of living persons at any given time who have had a stroke—depends on the interaction of incidence and survival. Studies in Rochester, Minnesota, have found stroke prevalence to be 500 to 800 cases per 100,000 population (Matsumoto, Whisnant, Kurland, et al., 1973; Whisnant, Fitzgibbons, Kurland, et al., 1971). These figures are similar to those of other countries (Terent, 1993).

Mortality

The average 30-day case fatality rate from stroke in the 1970s and 1980s was 21 percent, with a range from 17 percent (Broderick, Phillips,

Table 1. Epidemiology of stroke

Vital statistics—United States (1989)	
Incidence of stroke	500,000
Prevalence of stroke	2,980,000
Mortality due to stroke	147,470
Etiology of stroke (cerebral is used here to refer to the entire brain)[a]	
Ischemic stroke	**Percent**
Cerebral thrombosis	47–67
Cerebral embolus	14
Subtotal	61–81
Hemorrhagic stroke	
Intracerebral	8–16
Subarachnoid	4–8
Subtotal	12–24
Other or cause uncertain	0–25
Mortality rates (ranges from published reports)[b]	
30-day mortality	17–34
1-year mortality	25–40
3-year mortality	32–60
Risk factors for stroke[c]	
Potentially modifiable	**Not modifiable**
Transient ischemic attacks (TIA), especially in the presence of 70–99 percent carotid artery stenosis	Prior stroke
Hypertension	Age
Atrial fibrillation or other source of cardiac emboli	Race
Left ventricular hypertrophy	Gender
Congestive heart failure	Family history of stroke
Cigarette smoking	
Coronary artery disease	
Alcohol consumption	
Cocaine use	
Obesity	
Diabetes mellitus	
High serum cholesterol	

[a]Ranges reflect reports from four community-based studies (Bamford, Sandercock, Dennis, et al., 1990; Broderick, Phillips, Whisnant, et al., 1989; Kiyohara, Ueda, Hasuo, et al., 1989; Ward, Jamrozik, and Stewart-Wynne, 1988).
[b]Bonita, Beaglehole, and North, 1984; Broderick, Phillips, Whisnant, et al., 1989.
[c]Dyken, Wolf, Barnett, et al., 1984; Wolf, Cobb, and D'Agostino, 1992.

Note: The 1989 estimated incidence of stroke in the United States was 500,000; however, more recent data indicate that this estimate is closer to 550,000. For more information, see Prescott, 1994.

Whisnant, et al., 1989) to 34 percent (Bonita, Beaglehole, and North, 1984); 1-year mortality ranged from 25 to 40 percent; and 3-year mortality from 32 to 60 percent. Ten-year survival in the Framingham Study is 35 percent (Wolf, D'Agostino, O'Neal, et al., 1992). Hence, about half of the people with first strokes live for 3 or more years and more than one-third live for 10 years. Mortality rates for intracerebral hemorrhages are much higher than those for infarction. In Rochester (1984), the 30-day case fatality rate was 48 percent for intracerebral hemorrhage compared with 17 percent for all strokes (Broderick, Phillips, Whisnant, et al., 1989).

Stroke mortality rates have been declining steadily since the early 1950s in the United States (Broderick, Phillips, Whisnant, et al., 1989; Cooper, Sempos, Hsieh, et al., 1990) and most Western European countries (Bonita, Steward, and Beaglehole, 1990). The decline probably reflects the combined effects of better control of modifiable risk factors such as hypertension, earlier diagnosis, and better acute management of the patient (Broderick, Phillips, Whisnant, et al., 1989; Garraway, Whisnant, and Drury, 1983; McGovern, Burke, Sprafka, et al., 1992; Wolf, D'Agostino, O'Neal, et al., 1992).

Etiology

Stroke etiologies can be classified broadly into atherothrombotic brain infarction, hemorrhage, or other. A classification scheme for brain infarction (ischemic strokes) developed in the multicenter TOAST trial in the United States has the advantages of clinical relevance and reliability (Adams, Bendixen, Kappelle, et al., 1993). This system divides infarctions into large artery atherosclerosis, cardioembolism, small vessel occlusions, or infarcts of undetermined cause. Hemorrhages may be intracerebral or subarachnoid. Accurate diagnoses are difficult to achieve based on clinical impressions alone and require information from laboratory studies including computed tomography (CT) scanning, magnetic resonance imaging (MRI), and angiography. Even with laboratory studies, however, the diagnosis represents a "best clinical guess" in a substantial number of patients. Definitions differ among studies and need to be taken into account when interpreting the results.

Keeping in mind uncertainties about diagnostic accuracy, community-based studies report that 61 to 81 percent of first strokes represent infarctions, 8 to 16 percent intracerebral hemorrhages, and 4 to 8 percent subarachnoid hemorrhages (Broderick, Phillips, Whisnant, et al., 1989; Kiyohara, Ueda, Hasuo, et al., 1989; Oxfordshire Community Stroke Project, 1983; Ward, Jamrozik, and Steward-Wynne, 1988) (see Table 1). Accurate diagnosis is important because of the relationship of etiology to mortality, recurrence rates, and choice of treatment.

Risk Factors for Stroke

Risk factors for stroke can be divided into those that are potentially modifiable and those that are not (Dyken, Wolf, Barnett, et al., 1984). Most important among modifiable risk factors are TIAs, hypertension, diabetes mellitus, atrial fibrillation, left ventricular hypertrophy, and cigarette smoking. Prior stroke, age, sex, race, and family history are important nonmodifiable factors.

The paramount modifiable risk factor for stroke is hypertension. The relationship is with both diastolic and systolic blood pressure and is especially strong for levels above 160/95 mm Hg.

The presence of cardiac abnormalities such as atrial fibrillation, left ventricular hypertrophy, coronary heart disease, and congestive heart failure increases the risk of stroke at each blood pressure level. Acute myocardial infarction and atrial fibrillation predispose to embolism from cardiac thrombi, and nearly 15 percent of strokes in the Framingham Study have been attributed to atrial fibrillation (Wolf, Abbott, and Kannel, 1987). The risk of cerebral infarction is five times higher in individuals with electrocardiographic evidence of left ventricular hypertrophy even after other risk factors are taken into account. The relationship between blood lipids and stroke is not clear even though increased lipid levels have been related to carotid artery disease. Low serum cholesterol has been found in Hawaiian, Japanese, and other populations despite an increased incidence of cerebral hemorrhage (Yano, Reed, and MacLean, 1989).

The association of cigarette smoking with stroke holds for thrombotic strokes as well as intracerebral and subarachnoid hemorrhages. A recent meta-analysis of 32 studies found that smoking increased the risk of stroke by about 50 percent in both sexes and all age groups, and that risk was directly related to the number of cigarettes smoked per day (Shinton and Beevers, 1989).

Heavy consumption of alcohol, cocaine use, and obesity have also been linked to an increased incidence of stroke.

Among fixed risk factors, increasing age is by far the strongest. Seventy-two percent of strokes occur in people 65 years of age or over. Males have a higher risk of stroke than females in all but the oldest age groups, and African Americans have a twofold higher risk. In African Americans, about one-third of the increased risk is attributable to cardiovascular risk factors, another third to factors related to family income, and one-third is unexplained (Gillum, 1988).

Natural History of Recovery in Stroke Survivors

Neurological Deficits

Population-based studies provide the most reliable estimates of the relative frequency of neurological impairments following stroke. Even their results, however, need to be interpreted with knowledge of the time since stroke onset because of the importance of spontaneous neurological recovery during the early weeks after a stroke. Frequencies of deficits shortly after hospital admissions are provided by the Stroke Data Bank in the United States (Foulkes, Wolf, Price, et al., 1988; Sacco, unpublished data) and a stroke registry in Finland (Kotila, Waltimo, Niemi, et al., 1984); and frequencies of deficits 6 to 12 months (and longer) after strokes are provided by this same Finnish source and the Framingham Study (Gresham, Phillips, Wolf, et al., 1979). The Stroke Data Bank records data from admissions to four urban referral centers; the other two sources are population-based. The results are summarized in Table 2. The most striking findings are the large proportion of patients with hemiparesis and the high frequencies of other neurological deficits during the acute period, and the lower frequency of motor deficits, deficits in bladder control, dysphagia, dysarthria, and aphasia 6 to 12 months after stroke.

Table 2. Neurological deficits following stroke

	Acute		Chronic	
Neurological deficit	Stroke Data Bank[a] (infarctions only)	Finland[b]	Finland[b] (12 months)	Framingham[c] (6 or more months)
	Percent			
Right hemiparesis	44	NR	NR	22
Left hemiparesis	37	NR	NR	23
Bilateral hemiparesis	7	NR	NR	3
Total with hemiparesis	88	73	37	48
Ataxia	20	NR	NR	NR
Motor coordination	NR	86	61	NR
Hemianopsia	26	NR	NR	13
Visual-perceptual deficits	32	NR	41	NR
Aphasia	30	36	30	18
Dysarthria	48	57	21	16
Sensory deficits	53	NR	NR	24
Cognitive deficits (memory)	36	NR	(31)	NR
Depression	NR	NR	29	NR
Bladder control	29	29	9	NR
Dysphagia	12	13	4	NR

[a]From Sacco, unpublished data, and Foulkes, Wolf, Price, et al., 1988.
[b]From Kotila, Waltimo, Niemi, et al., 1984.
[c]From Gresham, Phillips, Wolf, et al., 1979.

Note: NR = not reported.

Comorbidities in Stroke Patients

Many patients have comorbid conditions that increase the risk of recurrent stroke and compromise the patient's ability to participate in active rehabilitation. The Framingham Study examined the frequency of comorbidities in stroke survivors and matched controls and found that the stroke survivors had significantly more hypertension (67 vs. 45 percent), hypertensive heart disease (53 vs. 31 percent), coronary heart disease (32 vs. 20 percent), obesity (22 vs. 12 percent), diabetes mellitus (22 vs. 10 percent), arthritis (22 vs. 12 percent), left ventricular hypertrophy (21 vs. 6 percent), and congestive heart failure (18 vs. 5 percent) (Gresham, Phillips, Wolf, et al., 1979).

Time Course of Recovery From Stroke

Neurological and functional recovery occurs most rapidly in the first 1 to 3 months after a stroke (Kelly-Hayes, Wolf, Kase, et al., 1989; Skilbeck, Wade, Hewer, et al., 1983), but some patients continue to progress after that time, especially with respect to language and visuospatial functions (Andrews, Brocklehurst, Richards, et al., 1981; Hier, Mondlock, and Caplan, 1983; Meerwaldt, 1983; Skilbeck, Wade, Hewer, et al., 1983). In Rochester, Minnesota, the proportion of patients with strokes who were "moderately severely" or "severely" disabled (Rankin grades IV or V) decreased from 58 percent at the time of stroke onset to 26 percent at discharge, and 17 percent among survivors after 6 months but remained relatively constant thereafter (Dombovy, Basford, Whisnant, et al., 1987). In Framingham, improvement in motor strength and performance of self-care functions slowed 3 months after stroke, but continued at a reduced pace throughout the first year, especially in patients with cerebral infarctions (Kelly-Hayes, Wolf, Kase, et al., 1989). Cognitive function improved only during the first 3 months. The Durham County Study (Duncan, 1992) found dramatic recovery of motor function during the first 30 days and slower but continued improvement thereafter in more severely impaired individuals. Arguments that neural and functional recovery can continue beyond 3 to 6 months are supported by a recent study in which patients with motor deficits were followed for 6 months after discharge from a rehabilitation unit (Ferruci, Bandinelli, Guralnik, et al., 1993). Though time since the onset of stroke was not reported, it is reasonable to assume that most patients were at least 2 months "poststroke" at the time of discharge. Neuromuscular function, mobility, and activities of daily living continued to improve during followup, especially in more severely impaired patients.

Disability After Stroke

Mobility. Mobility problems are common during the acute stroke period, but a large majority of survivors are able to walk with or without assistance 6 months to a year later. Only 27 percent of enrollees in the Frenchay Health District Stroke Registry were able to walk independently during the first week after their strokes, but 85 percent were able to do so after 6 months (Wade and Hewer, 1987a). Seventy-eight percent of long-term stroke survivors in the Framingham Study were able to walk (Gresham, Phillips, Wolf, et al., 1979).

Activities of Daily Living. "Basic" activities of daily living (ADL) include mobility and self-care functions such as dressing, bathing, feeding, toileting, grooming, and transfers (e.g., chair to bed, in and out of bath) that a person must be able to perform to be independent. "Instrumental" activities of daily living (IADL) are more complex functions such as use of a telephone, meal preparation, money management, use of public transportation, home and child-care tasks, and recreational and work activities. Basic ADL is usually measured on disability scales such as those recommended in Chapter 3. Findings from population-based studies (Dombovy, 1993) indicate that independence in self-care ADL improves with time. Partial or total dependence in self-care ADL was reported in 67 to 88 percent of patients within 3 weeks of onset of stroke (Dombovy, Basford, Whisnant, et al., 1987; Kojima, Omura, Wakamatsu, et al., 1990; Kotila, Waltimo, Niemi, et al., 1984; Wade and Hewer, 1987a), but in only 24 to 53 percent of survivors 6 months to 5 years after their strokes (Ahlsio, Britton, Murray, et al., 1984; Dombovy, Basford, Whisnant, et al., 1987; Gresham, Phillips, Wolf, et al., 1979; Kojima, Omura, Wakamatsu, et al., 1990; Kotila, Waltimo, Niemi, et al., 1984; Wade and Hewer, 1987a). The exclusion of fatalities needs to be considered in interpreting long-term results since these individuals usually have had more severe strokes. Frequencies and recovery patterns for different types of ADL in a community study in the United Kingdom are shown in Table 3.

Communication. The ability to communicate is important both for successful participation in rehabilitation and for resumption of an independent life. Patients with communication deficits usually experience some degree of spontaneous improvement. One study, for example, found that the frequency of aphasia decreased from 24 percent within 7 days after stroke (with another 28 percent unassessable) to 12 percent 6 months later (Wade, Hewer, David, et al., 1986). Formal assessment may underestimate the true frequency of communication deficits, however, since 44 percent of patients and 57 percent of caregivers in this study thought speech was abnormal at the time of followup.

Neuropsychological Functioning. Neuropsychological disabilities can be divided broadly into cognitive dysfunction, visuospatial deficits, and affective disorders (predominantly depression). Depression is particularly common after stroke. In Finland, Kotila found depression in 44 percent of

Table 3. Disabilities after stroke in the Frenchay Health District, United Kingdom, during 1981-1983

Type of disability	Acute[a]	6 months
	Percent	
Not oriented	55	27
Marked communication problem	52	15
Motor loss (partial or complete)	80	53
Bowel incontinence	31	7
Urinary incontinence	44	11
Needs help with grooming	56	13
Needs help with toileting	68	20
Needs help with feeding	68	33
Needs help with dressing	79	31
Needs help with bathing	86	49
Needs help with transfers from bed to chair	70	19
Unable to walk independently	73	15
Very severely dependent	38	4
Severely dependent	20	5
Moderately dependent	15	12
Mildly dependent	12	32
Physically independent	12	47

[a]Acute figures are minimal estimates for acute stroke, since many patients were not assessed during the first week after onset.

Source: Adapted with permission from Wade, 1994.

patients and other abnormal emotional reactions in 30 percent of patients 3 months after stroke, and corresponding figures of 29 and 32 percent 12 months after stroke (Kotila, Waltimo, Niemi, et al., 1984).

Quality of Life After Stroke

Most stroke survivors experience a decrease in levels of activity and overall quality of life. In the Framingham Study, they were found to socialize less, have fewer interests and hobbies, be less able to use public transportation or perform household tasks, and be less likely to engage in vocational pursuits than a stroke-free control group (Gresham, Phillips, Wolf, et al., 1979). In another study, they consistently reported that their quality of life was worse than before the stroke and had not improved over the 2 intervening years (Ahlsio, Britton, Murray, et al., 1984). In this study, deterioration was at least as strongly related to psychological problems such as depression and anxiety as to physical dependency measured by ADL. Depression, dependence on others, and inability to return to work all contribute to diminished quality of life (Niemi, Laaksonen, Kotila, et al., 1988; Viitanen, Fugl-Meyer, Bernspang, et al., 1988).

The ability to return home is also an important dimension of the quality of life, though the resulting burden on caregivers may offset the benefits. Rates of institutionalization after stroke range from 10 to 29 percent (Dombovy, Basford, Whisnant, et al., 1987; Gresham, Phillips, Wolf, et al., 1979; Kelly-Hayes, Wolf, Kannel, et al., 1988; Kotila, Waltimo, Niemi, et al., 1984; Lehmann, DeLateur, Fowler, et al., 1975; Silliman, Wagner, and Fletcher, 1987).

Gender Differences

Age-adjusted disability levels after stroke are similar in men and women (Wade, Hewer, David, et al., 1986). However, women report more disability and unmet social needs (Branch and Jette, 1981; Jette and Branch, 1981). Greater differences have been found in women between actual lifestyles and observed capacity to function (Kelly-Hayes, Jette, Wolf, et al., 1992). In Framingham, women are institutionalized twice as often as men (Kelly-Hayes, Wolf, Kannel, et al., 1988). Marital status is a more important predictor of the patient's ability to live independently in men than in women, due at least partly to the greater support provided by female caregivers (DeJong and Branch, 1982).

Prediction of Functional Recovery After Stroke

A special report from the World Health Organization (1989) succinctly states the problem of predicting which patients will benefit from rehabilitation:

> *Since rehabilitation can be costly, the development of improved criteria for selecting patients for intensive rehabilitation is of the utmost importance. Such selection should be based on the prognosis of the recovery of function(s) in three main groups: (1) patients who spontaneously make good recovery without rehabilitation; (2) patients who can make satisfactory recovery only through intensive rehabilitation; and (3) patients with poor recovery of function irrespective of the type of rehabilitation.* (p. 1429)

Available evidence does not permit a clear delineation among these three groups of patients. Controlled clinical trials are needed to identify who is most likely to benefit from rehabilitation. Until these studies are performed, clinicians must rely on observational studies to estimate the effects of different patient characteristics on functional recovery. These studies do not, however, differentiate the benefits of rehabilitation from spontaneous recovery.

In more than a single study, patient characteristics that have been associated with poorer functional outcomes include severe initial functional deficits, severe initial motor deficits, persistent urinary incontinence, severe visuospatial deficits, sitting imbalance, severe aphasia, altered level of consciousness, severe cognitive deficits, major depression, severe comorbidities, disability prior to stroke, and older age. Despite their limitations, these results provide a useful starting point for identifying subgroups of stroke survivors who are likely to fall in Category 3 as defined by WHO, and in whom the potential benefits of stroke rehabilitation need to be carefully evaluated.

3 Assessment Methods for Patients With Strokes

Introduction

Objectives of assessment are to:

- Document the diagnosis of stroke, its etiology, area of the brain involved, and clinical manifestations.
- Identify treatment needs during the acute phase.
- Identify patients who are most likely to benefit from rehabilitation.
- Select the appropriate type of rehabilitation setting.
- Provide the basis for creating a rehabilitation treatment plan.
- Monitor progress during rehabilitation and facilitate discharge planning.
- Monitor progress after return to a community residence.

To achieve these objectives, assessments must be performed by people skilled in rehabilitation, using a combination of clinical examinations and well-validated standardized measures. A battery of instruments is often required because of the varied clinical manifestations of stroke. Also, the goals of assessment change over the clinical course of stroke—from initial concern with survival, level of consciousness, and responses to acute treatments—to a later focus on specific neurological impairments and, during and after rehabilitation, on functional abilities. Measurement is affected by the complex relationships among deficits, impairments, and disabilities; e.g., a patient's inability to propel a wheelchair independently could result from any combination of the following factors: motor weakness, impaired cognition, communication problems, perceptual deficits, sensorimotor deficits, limited cardiovascular endurance, or lack of motivation. Environmental factors may also contribute to the patient's disability (e.g., there could be a defect in the wheelchair or an access impediment).

At present, assessment practices vary widely, and no single measure or group of measures has been universally accepted. Numerous measures are in use, but only a few of these have been adequately validated. Also, many clinicians have been reluctant to adopt standardized instruments. Reports that formal assessments may be more reliable than clinical impressions may help to overcome this resistance (Tinetti, 1986).

In recommending assessment instruments, this guideline attempts to balance validity and comprehensiveness of assessment with practicality. It also recognizes that there may be no single *best* method or instrument within each domain and, in most cases, suggests several options. Attachments 1 to 13 at the end of this guideline provide tables listing recommended assessment instruments for patients with stroke. The tables briefly describe each instrument and provide information on how the instrument is used, the time required to administer it, and its principal strengths and weaknesses.

The strengths and limitations of a wide variety of assessment instruments are carefully analyzed in *Measurement in Neurological Rehabilitation* (Wade, 1992). This book is an invaluable reference for those interested in improving the treatment of post-stroke patients.

Stages of Assessment

The principal stages of assessment in stroke rehabilitation are summarized in Figure 3. Additional examinations may be dictated by the needs of particular patients.

Assessment begins with a clinical evaluation at the time of admission to the acute care hospital. Subsequent examinations during the acute hospitalization document changes in neurological and medical status and responses to treatment. Screening for post-stroke rehabilitation is performed when the patient is medically and neurologically stable. On the basis of the screening, the patient may be referred to an interdisciplinary rehabilitation program or to individual rehabilitation services in an ambulatory setting, or the decision may be not to recommend rehabilitation at that time.

A detailed assessment is performed at the time of admission to a rehabilitation program to validate the appropriateness of the referral, formulate treatment goals and a rehabilitation management plan, and provide a baseline for monitoring progress. Periodic reassessment during rehabilitation documents progress and provides the information needed to adjust treatment and eventually to plan for discharge or transfer to another type of rehabilitation setting. After discharge from rehabilitation, assessment is performed to monitor adaptation to a community residence and maintenance of functional gains made during rehabilitation.

The content of assessment at each stage is discussed at its chronologic place in the course of treatment for stroke in Chapters 4 to 7. The focus of the present chapter is on assessment methods and measures.

Criteria for Evaluating Assessment Instruments

The essential characteristics on which clinical assessment instruments are evaluated are sensibility, validity, reliability, and sensitivity to change.

- **Sensibility** refers to the instrument's overall reasonableness, importance, and ease of use. Feinstein (1987) suggests that sensibility is the major factor determining the success or failure of a clinical measure.
- **Validity** is the ability of an instrument to measure what it is intended and presumed to measure. An instrument's **criterion validity** is determined by comparing its results to an agreed-on *gold standard*. Its **predictive validity** is its ability to predict future outcomes.

Figure 3. Stages of assessment for post-stroke rehabilitation

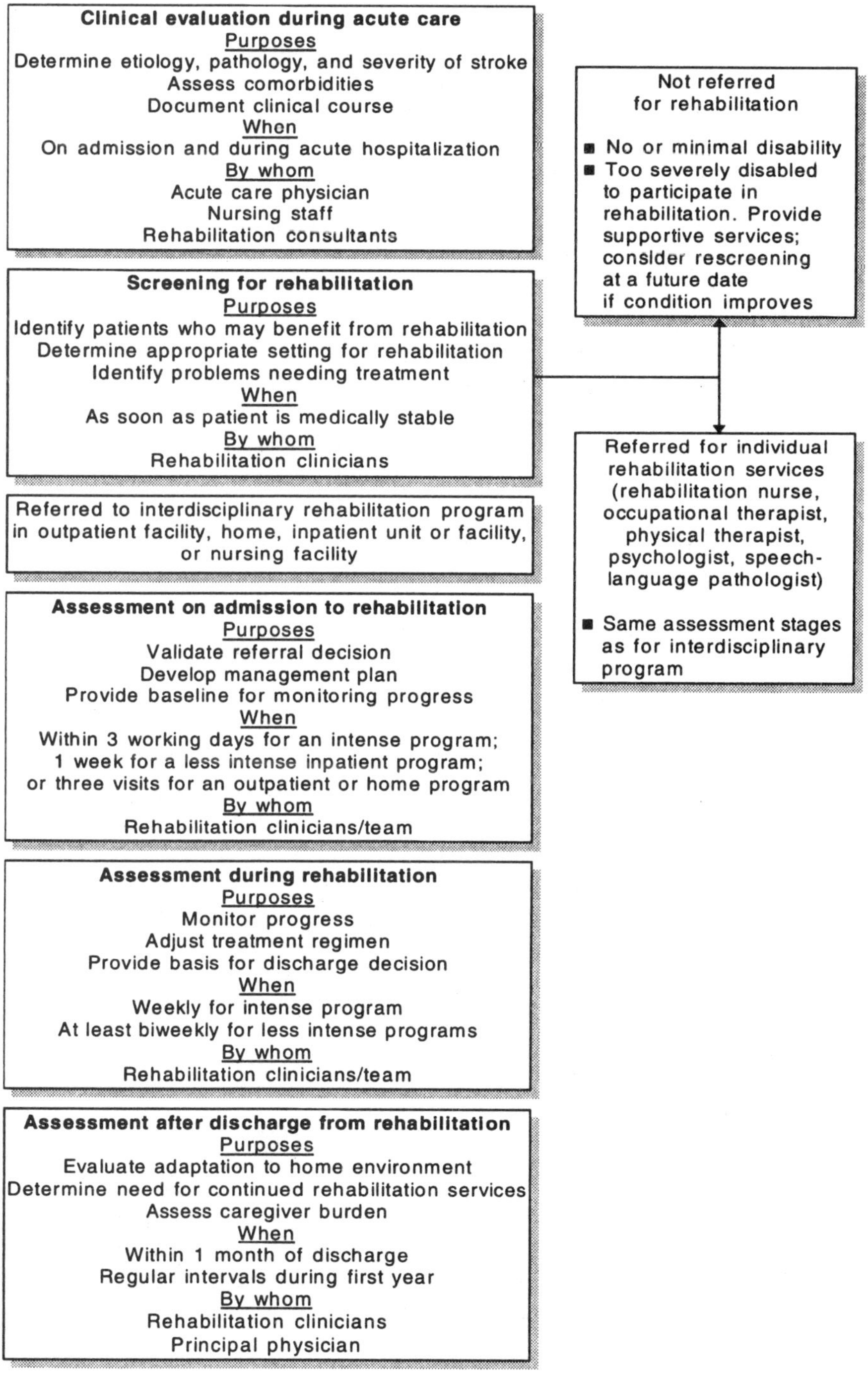

Clinical evaluation during acute care
Purposes
Determine etiology, pathology, and severity of stroke
Assess comorbidities
Document clinical course
When
On admission and during acute hospitalization
By whom
Acute care physician
Nursing staff
Rehabilitation consultants

Screening for rehabilitation
Purposes
Identify patients who may benefit from rehabilitation
Determine appropriate setting for rehabilitation
Identify problems needing treatment
When
As soon as patient is medically stable
By whom
Rehabilitation clinicians

Not referred for rehabilitation

- No or minimal disability
- Too severely disabled to participate in rehabilitation. Provide supportive services; consider rescreening at a future date if condition improves

Referred for individual rehabilitation services (rehabilitation nurse, occupational therapist, physical therapist, psychologist, speech-language pathologist)

- Same assessment stages as for interdisciplinary program

Referred to interdisciplinary rehabilitation program in outpatient facility, home, inpatient unit or facility, or nursing facility

Assessment on admission to rehabilitation
Purposes
Validate referral decision
Develop management plan
Provide baseline for monitoring progress
When
Within 3 working days for an intense program;
1 week for a less intense inpatient program;
or three visits for an outpatient or home program
By whom
Rehabilitation clinicians/team

Assessment during rehabilitation
Purposes
Monitor progress
Adjust treatment regimen
Provide basis for discharge decision
When
Weekly for intense program
At least biweekly for less intense programs
By whom
Rehabilitation clinicians/team

Assessment after discharge from rehabilitation
Purposes
Evaluate adaptation to home environment
Determine need for continued rehabilitation services
Assess caregiver burden
When
Within 1 month of discharge
Regular intervals during first year
By whom
Rehabilitation clinicians
Principal physician

- **Reliability** has two dimensions. **Interobserver reliability** refers to the ability of two different individuals who administer the instrument to a particular patient to achieve similar results. **Test-retest reliability** refers to whether repeated use of the measure yields consistent results in the absence of a change in the patient.
- **Sensitivity to change** is the ability of the measure to detect clinically important changes. Instruments used to monitor the patient's progress during rehabilitation must accommodate the full range of performance levels, must have scales with sufficiently fine gradations that small changes can be detected, and must permit evaluation of specific types of impairments or disabilities rather than relying solely on summary scores.

The instruments recommended in this guideline are in wide use and have been evaluated with respect to most or all of the above criteria. They are practical and feasible to administer, and they yield meaningful results that can easily be communicated to the patient and family.

The Neurological Examination

Neurological findings that most strongly influence rehabilitation decisions are summarized in Table 4. The reader should consult a standard text for a complete discussion of the neurological examination.

Level of Consciousness

Disturbances in consciousness are a strong predictor of adverse outcomes after stroke. They are more likely when brain damage is extensive, especially if the brain stem is involved or when cerebral edema or increased intracranial pressure is present. A prolonged deep coma after a stroke is rare and is more likely to complicate intracranial hemorrhage than infarction.

Evaluation of the level of consciousness involves observation of the patient's spontaneous behavior, responses to external stimuli (verbal or painful), and interactions with others. It is usually described in terms of the patient's best performance as being alert, drowsy, stuporous, or comatose. Repeated observations are needed because findings often fluctuate.

Cognitive Disorders

Disorders in higher brain functions are common after stroke. The full picture of dementia is rare after a first event but does occur as a result of multiple strokes. A general impression of memory and the ability to acquire and retain new information can be obtained from observation of the patient's interactions with other persons and from observation of responses to questions on: orientation (name, place, day of week, etc.), current events, recent personal history, arithmetic, and simple tests of recall. Additional testing with a mental status screening test (discussed

Table 4. Selected results of the neurological examination

Type of deficit	Component examination	Key findings	Effect of persistent deficit on rehabilitation
Altered level of consciousness	Repeated observation and testing of responses to external stimuli. Glasgow Coma Scale.	Drowsy, stuporous, comatose.	An altered level of consciousness is a contraindication to rehabilitation.
Cognitive deficits in higher functions, memory, ability to learn	Observation; questions to probe mental functions; standardized screening test.	Degrees and types of deficits.	A severe deficit is a contraindication to rehabilitation; a moderate deficit may impede rehabilitation and needs to be incorporated into the rehabilitation management plan.
Motor deficits	Tests of strength and tone in muscles of the upper and lower extremity and face.	Degree(s) and site(s) of weakness, incoordination, abnormal movements.	Motor deficits are the primary indications for rehabilitation. Absence of any voluntary movement is a poor prognostic sign.
Disturbances in balance and coordination	Tests of coordination, sitting, standing, walking.	Degree(s) and type(s) of deficits.	Deficits impede but do not contraindicate rehabilitation.
Somatosensory deficits	Specific tests for sensory modalities (pain, touch, etc.); complex sensory tests.	Degree(s) and type(s) of deficits.	Deficits impede but do not contraindicate rehabilitation.
Disorders of vision	Pupillary responses, ocular motility, optic fundus exam, visual fields and acuity.	Visual loss or field defect; conjugate gaze deficits.	Severe visual loss or ocular motility disturbances will impede rehabilitation.
Unilateral neglect	Observation; describe complex picture; sensory testing.	One side of body or external environment ignored; often clears spontaneously.	Neglect impedes rehabilitation but is not a contraindication.

Table 4. Selected results of the neurological examination (continued)

Type of deficit	Component examination	Key findings	Effect of persistent deficit on rehabilitation
Speech and language deficits	Observation of spontaneous speech and language use; including language comprehension, and if possible, simple reading and writing skills.	Aphasia, dysarthrias, or apraxias of speech.	Severe problems in communication will impede rehabilitation. Treatment becomes an integral part of rehabilitation.
Swallowing disorder (dysphagia)	History; test of ability to swallow liquids and solids; cinefluoroscopy with barium swallow.	Abnormal swallowing mechanism, aspiration.	Dysphagia requires careful attention to avoid aspiration and pneumonia.
Affective disorders	History; observation; depression screening test.	Symptoms of depression.	Depression may impede rehabilitation, if not treated.
Pain	Description of pain by patient; observation of restrictions in range of motion; observation of facial expressions or resistance to movement.	Location and severity of pain; precipitating causes.	Pain may require specific treatment or medication. It impedes rehabilitation.

later) or a neuropsychological examination is needed to define cognitive or behavioral deficits more fully. Care must be taken to distinguish cognitive deficits from difficulties in communication.

Moderate to severe higher level cognitive deficits will markedly interfere with learning new skills during rehabilitation.

Motor Deficits

The nature and severity of motor deficits reflect the type, location, and extent of the vascular lesion. Motor deficits can occur in isolation or may be accompanied by sensory, cognitive, or speech deficits. Weakness and paralysis are the most common manifestations, but incoordination, clumsiness, involuntary movements, or abnormal postures also occur. The face, upper extremity, and lower extremity can be involved alone or in combination. Common patterns are hemiparesis (one arm and leg) and monoparesis (most commonly the upper extremity). Patients may also demonstrate apraxias of movements in which the individual does not have demonstrable muscle weakness but is unable to sequence movement patterns. Motor limitations may be subtle in some patients.

The position of involved limbs at rest and spontaneous limb movements should be noted and the strength of muscles recorded using a scale such as: grade 0 = no movement, 1 = palpable contraction or flicker, 2 = contraction with gravity eliminated, 3 = movement against gravity, 4 = movement against resistance but weaker than other side, and 5 = normal strength. Increased (spasticity) or decreased (flaccidity) muscle tone can be identified from the degree of resistance felt to rapid passive limb movement. Slow movements (bradykinesia) or motor abnormalities such as chorea, athetosis, or hemiballismus should be recorded. Examinations for abnormal muscle stretch reflexes or pathologic reflexes are traditional, but their presence does not predict recovery from stroke. The ability to walk and to perform skilled movements (e.g., handwriting or the use of utensils) also needs to be tested; standard instruments to aid in these assessments are discussed later.

Most patients experience some spontaneous improvement in motor deficits, but the degree of recovery varies widely. Persistent motor deficits are often the primary indication for rehabilitation because of their influence on the performance of daily activities.

Disturbances in Balance and Coordination

Motor or sensory deficits and dysfunction of the cerebellum or vestibular system can produce disturbances in balance or coordination. Incoordination in the absence of motor or sensory loss is known as ataxia. Disturbances in coordination can be examined at the bedside by performing finger-to-nose, heel-to-shin, and alternating movement tests. When possible, the patient's ability to stand and walk should be tested. If a patient can walk, additional examinations such as tandem walking or the Romberg test can provide helpful information.

Somatosensory Deficits

Somatosensory deficits can range from the loss of simple sensory modalities to complex sensory disorders. Patients complain of numbness, tingling, or abnormal sensations (dysesthesia), or they show excessive reactions to sensory stimuli (hyperesthesia). Interactions may occur between cognitive and somatosensory disturbances. The sensory examination is difficult to perform and may be unreliable in the confused or cognitively impaired patient. The bedside examination involves testing sensory modalities such as pain, temperature, touch, proprioception (sense of position), kinesthesia (sense of movement), and pallesthesia (sense of vibration). Complex somatic sensory testing includes stereognosis and graphesthesia.

Sensory deficits usually improve after stroke, although some residual loss is common. Profound sensory loss will hamper rehabilitation of motor impairments.

Disorders of Vision

Stroke can cause visual deficits, most commonly homonymous hemianopsia. Examination of pupillary responses and ocular motility, direct observation of the ocular fundus, and measurement of corrected visual acuity and visual fields are important. A visual-field defect in the nondominant field needs to be differentiated from visual neglect since the latter often improves spontaneously, while visual-field defects usually do not improve. Stroke can also lead to complex visual deficits or disturbances in color vision. Paralysis of conjugate gaze is an unfavorable prognostic sign for survival but usually improves spontaneously in survivors. Ocular motility disturbances due to brain stem strokes may produce symptoms such as diplopia, vertigo, oscillopsia, or visual distortions. Severe visual disturbances will increase the complexity of rehabilitation.

Unilateral Neglect

Neglect refers to a patient's lack of awareness of a specific part of the body or external environment and occurs primarily in nondominant (usually right) hemisphere strokes. In these patients, sensory stimuli (vision, hearing, somatosensory) in the left half of the environment are ignored or evoke muted responses. Severely afflicted patients will deny problems or illness or may not even recognize their own body parts. Bedside evaluation will find that the patient is turned to the right and will often not turn toward an observer on the left. Testing will demonstrate that the patient ignores items in the left visual field when asked to describe a complex picture and ignores sensory stimuli on the left. Neglect usually improves spontaneously and relatively quickly, but it will significantly complicate rehabilitation while it persists.

Speech and Language Deficits

Aphasia is frequent after vascular events in the language-dominant hemisphere and may cause disturbances in comprehension, speech, verbal expression, reading, and writing. Bedside evaluation includes naming of objects and observing patterns of fluency, adequacy of content, prosody of speech, use of grammatical forms, ability to repeat, and comprehension of spoken language. If possible, rudimentary writing and reading should be observed.

Neuromotor disturbances (dysarthria and apraxia of speech) need to be differentiated from aphasia. Dysarthria may be due to dysfunction of the larynx, pharynx, palate, tongue, lips, or mouth. It causes difficulty in making speech sounds clearly, abnormalities in prosody, or changes in voice quality. Observation of spontaneous speech needs to be supplemented by asking the patient to say words or phrases that test specific parts of the articulatory mechanism. In apraxia of speech, the patient is unable to program a sequence of volitional movements despite the absence of motor deficits. This results in difficulty in initiating speech, inconsistent speech patterns, and difficulty in positioning the articulatory mechanism for complex speech movements.

Apraxia of speech, dysarthria, and aphasia frequently coexist. Proper management depends on the ability to differentiate among the three conditions and determine the relative contributions of each to a patient's overall speech disorder. Language patterns and speech disturbances frequently improve during recovery from stroke.

Pain

Severe headache, neck pain, or face pain can result from either hemorrhagic or ischemic stroke. Pain can also be associated with complications of stroke such as adhesive capsulitis; a rotator cuff tear in the shoulder; reflex sympathetic dystrophy; entrapment of the ulnar, median, or peroneal nerves; decubitus ulcer; or contractures. Neurogenic pain after stroke is a particularly serious problem. This syndrome most commonly occurs with strokes involving the thalamus. It may not appear until weeks or months after the stroke's onset. It usually involves the contralateral half of the body and may be intense and relentless. On examination, patients will be very sensitive to touch. Spontaneous recovery is rare. Pain of any cause can greatly impede a patient's ability to participate in rehabilitation and may require treatment with medications, surgical procedures, or nerve blocks.

Diagnostic Tests

Diagnostic tests are used to supplement the patient's medical history and neurological and physical examinations in order to (1) confirm the diagnosis of stroke; (2) determine its cause (subarachnoid or intracerebral hemorrhage, embolism or thrombosis), location in the brain, and extent; (3) evaluate complications of stroke and cardiovascular and other comorbid diseases that will influence treatment or clinical outcomes; and (4) assess risk factors for recurrent stroke. Test results may have an important influence on treatment decisions during acute care and on assessment of needs for rehabilitation.

Some tests, such as CT of the brain, electrocardiogram, echocardiogram, coagulation studies, complete blood count, and blood glucose, are obtained on admission because their results may influence initial management. Other studies, such as MRI, cerebral arteriography, or cerebral spinal fluid examination, may be performed for specific indications to verify the etiology of stroke or assess changes in the patient's condition. Discussion of the indications for specific diagnostic tests is beyond the scope of this guideline.

Assessment of Comorbid Diseases

Comorbid neurological or medical diseases may affect recovery from a stroke and limit or contraindicate specific treatments or rehabilitation. Important conditions are cardiovascular diseases (ischemic heart disease, congestive heart failure, hypertension), chronic pulmonary diseases (asthma, bronchitis, emphysema), diabetes mellitus, cancer, musculoskeletal diseases (arthritis, amputations, orthopedic problems), severe psychiatric diseases, and neurological diseases (Alzheimer's or Parkinson's disease). The evaluation of these conditions is beyond the scope of this guideline.

Assessment of Functional Health Patterns

Assessment and continuous monitoring of basic health functions are important throughout the acute care of stroke and stroke rehabilitation. Special attention should be directed to vital signs (blood pressure, heart rate, temperature, and respiration), swallowing disorders, nutrition and hydration, bowel and bladder function, skin integrity, physical activity endurance, and sleep patterns. Goals are to prevent complications or identify them early in their development so that treatment can be given and additional disability avoided.

Swallowing disorders (dysphagia) may occur due to dysfunction of the lips, mouth, tongue, palate, pharynx, larynx, or proximal esophagus. Deficits can occur in any phase of swallowing, from the oral preparatory phase to the esophageal phase. Early assessment and treatment help to prevent aspiration and dehydration or malnutrition from inadequate oral intake. Aspiration into the airway may occur before a swallow due to disordered tongue function or a delayed or absent triggering of the swallowing mechanism; during swallowing from reduced laryngeal elevation; or after swallowing as a result of residue in the pharynx, reduced pharyngeal peristalsis, or diverticulum formation (Logemann, 1986).

Assessment includes careful pharyngeal and laryngeal nerve examinations and testing of facial muscles, tongue function, and the cough response (DiIorio and Price, 1990). Observation during eating may reveal that the patient dribbles from the mouth, pockets food on one side of the mouth, coughs or chokes when swallowing, drains food or liquid from the nose, holds food in the back of the mouth for long periods, or complains of nasal burning or tickling in the throat (Emick-Herring and Wood, 1990). The quality of the patient's voice may be affected and dysphonia (wet, hoarse voice) may be noted. Videofluoroscopy using a modified barium swallow method can be used to evaluate swallowing time, pharyngeal motility, and the mechanism of aspiration (Chen, Ott, Peele, et al., 1990; Horner and Massey, 1988; Horner, Massey, Riski, et al., 1988; Linden and Siebens, 1983; Logemann, 1986; Veis and Logemann, 1985).

Adequate **nutrition** and **hydration** can be compromised by altered consciousness, dysphagia, sensory or perceptual deficits, reduced mobility, or depression, which can cause decreased interest in eating. Poor hydration or metabolic imbalance, in turn, contributes to the development of infections, pressure sores, confusion, and poor physical endurance. Assessment includes monitoring intake, body weight, urinary and fecal outputs, caloric counts, levels of serum proteins, electrolytes, and blood counts (Axelsson, Asplund, Norberg, et al., 1988).

Disturbances of **bladder** or **bowel function** are often seen. Urinary incontinence can result from inattention, mental status changes, immobility, bladder hyperreflexia or hyporeflexia, disturbances of sphincter control, or sensory loss. Persistent incontinence should be evaluated to identify treatable medical conditions such as urinary tract infections and to determine needs for external drainage or nursing measures to maintain cleanliness and prevent skin breakdown.

Alterations in bowel function can manifest either as incontinence and diarrhea or as constipation and impaction; the latter is far more common. Assessment of constipation includes careful documentation of past and present bowel habits, dietary and fluid intake, and activity.

Skin breakdown is more likely in patients with incontinence, infections, and limited mobility (Clarke and Kadhom, 1988; Gerson, 1975; [AHCPR-sponsored] Panel for the Prediction and Prevention of Pressure Ulcers in Adults, 1992). Abnormal movement patterns, sensory deficits, and nutritional depletion compound the risk. Daily examination of the patient's skin, especially over pressure points, is the key to assessment. Assessment tools to aid in documenting and preventing pressure ulcers include the Braden Scale (Bergstrom, Braden, Laguzza, et al., 1987; Bergstrom, Demuth, and Braden, 1987; Braden, 1989; Braden and Bergstrom, 1987 and 1992) and the Norton Scale (Norton, McLaren, and Exton-Smith, 1962).

A patient's **physical activity endurance** may be insufficient for performing ADL (Mol and Baker, 1991). Potentially treatable causes, such as deconditioning as a result of immobilization and cardiovascular diseases, need to be carefully evaluated. Physical activity endurance is especially important because of its influence on the pace and intensity of rehabilitation. There is no standard approach used by rehabilitation programs to evaluate physical activity endurance. Observation of symptoms during exercise; ease of fatigability; responses of blood pressure, heart rate, and rhythm; and respiration to exercise are important dimensions. Submaximal exercise stress tests are useful in suitable patients.

Disturbances of **sleep patterns** are common and may persist for months after a stroke. They may lead to sluggish responses that can be confused with lack of interest, lack of motivation, or depression. Sleep patterns throughout the day and night need to be carefully observed and documented.

Assessment of Depression and Other Affective Disorders

Depression is common after stroke. The most effective means of diagnosis is a clinical interview administered by a knowledgeable mental health professional. This interview should include questions about common symptoms, their severity, and their time course. The patient's mental status and communicative abilities should be examined simultaneously so that symptoms can be interpreted in context. Assessment may be especially difficult in patients with aphasia or severe comprehension deficits. Complex situations may require intensive investigation that takes behavioral observation of the patient, self-reports, and family reports (Gordon, 1992; Hibbard, Gordon, Stein, et al., 1993). Standardized depression scales may be useful in screening for depressive symptoms and monitoring responses to treatment, but should not be relied on as the only basis for the diagnosis of depression.

Other emotional or behavioral disturbances (e.g., anxiety, mania, outbursts of uncontrolled behavior, emotionless affect, and hostility) also occur in patients with stroke but are much less common than depression. Each depends on the clinical interview for diagnosis.

Assessment of Neuropsychological Function

Cognitive impairments detected on neurological examination or a mental status screening test warrant a thorough clinical evaluation by a mental health professional and, in selected patients, comprehensive neuropsychological testing.

Commonly used tests are shown in Table 5. Some of these tests represent batteries of subtests that tap several areas of cognition, while others examine only a single domain. The selection of tests or test batteries for a specific patient is complex and should be made by a trained neuropsychologist. This guideline does not address selection criteria or recommend any specific tests.

Assessment of Family Functioning and Other Contextual Factors

Contextual factors, especially family structure and functioning, are important throughout rehabilitation, but become particularly critical during discharge planning and after return to a community living environment.

Table 5. Frequently used neuropsychological tests

Frequently used neuropsychological tests
Intelligence tests ■ Wechsler Adult Intelligence Scale (WAIS) ■ Peabody Picture Vocabulary Test (Revised)
Memory tests ■ Wechsler Memory Scale Revised (WMS-R) ■ Wechsler Memory Scale (WMS) ■ Rey Auditory Verbal Learning
Language tests ■ Boston Naming Test ■ Multilingual Aphasia Exam Subtests (Token Test, Controlled Oral Word Association)
Visuospatial tests ■ Rey-Osterrieth Complex Figure ■ Rey-Osterrieth Delayed Recall ■ Raven's Progressive Matrices
Executive "higher order" measures ■ Wisconsin Card Sorting
Executive "mental control" measures ■ Stroop Color-Word Test
Benton test ■ Benton Visual Retention Test ■ Benton Judgment of Line Orientation
Achievement tests ■ Wide-Range Achievement Test
Neuropsychological batteries ■ Halstead-Reitan Battery ■ Subtests (Trails A, Trails B, Finger Tapping)
Psychomotor functioning ■ Grooved Pegboard
Personality tests ■ Minnesota Multiphasic ■ Personality Inventory (MMPI)

Contextual factors pertaining to the patient, family or other caregivers, living environment, and community are summarized in Table 6. Important contextual factors include:

- Presence of a spouse or significant other.
- Whether the patient was living with family members before the stroke.
- Family members who can supply support, and their ages and health.
- Family members within reasonable distance of the patient.

Table 6. Important contextual factors in the patient with a stroke

Patient characteristics ■ Demographics (age, gender, race, ethnicity, language, education). ■ History of mental illness. ■ Personal life and work history. ■ Prior activity level (low to very high). ■ Prior socialization (isolated to outgoing). ■ Previous coping strategies. ■ Preferred leisure activities and hobbies. ■ Participation in social programs during rehabilitation. ■ Expectations regarding stroke outcomes and need for assistance. ■ Ability to mobilize support.
Family and caregiver characteristics ■ Demographics (age, gender, race, ethnicity, language, education). ■ Members of household and relationship to patient. ■ Current developmental stage of family (young children, empty nest, retired). ■ Other family members within reasonable distance. ■ Other potential caregivers. ■ Family history of medical or mental illness; alcohol or substance abuse. ■ Family's structure and functioning. ■ Family patterns of socialization. ■ Capacity to provide physical, emotional, instrumental support. ■ Family's coping and adaptation patterns (previous crises and responses). ■ Ability to mobilize supports. ■ Attitudes toward illness, treatment, and disability. ■ Cultural beliefs and norms likely to influence responses to rehabilitation. ■ Family occupations, income, and financial resources. ■ Health insurance.
Living environment and community characteristics ■ Access to building and key facilities within living quarters. ■ Safety considerations. ■ Access to resources and activities in community. ■ Level of stimulation in home and community.
Institutions and agencies ■ Prior membership or contacts with churches, synagogues, schools, special interest groups, etc. ■ Availability of potentially needed resources in the community. ■ Availability of health care and rehabilitation facilities. ■ Home care agencies. ■ Previous workplace.

- Family history (of medical, mental health, alcohol, or drug abuse problems).
- Family ethnicity and native language.
- Physical environment of potential residences.

Information is obtained by interviewing the patient and family.

Recommended Standardized Assessment Instruments

Information from standardized assessment instruments complements that from the neurological examination in assessing the level of consciousness, the overall extent of neurological impairment, motor function, balance, cognition, and speech and language. Standardized instruments also facilitate evaluation of the patient's actual performance of activities such as walking and basic or instrumental activities of daily living (ADL and IADL). These are a useful adjunct to the clinical interview in assessing depression, and they can help to apply objective measures to the elusive factors of family functioning and quality of life. Good test-retest and interobserver reliability of standardized instruments is particularly valuable in monitoring a patient's progress and in assessing performance of a rehabilitation program over time.

Overall Measures of Stroke Deficits

The Glasgow Coma Scale (see Attachment 1) provides a systematic way to monitor changes in the level of consciousness.

Stroke deficit scales (see Attachment 2) provide a quick, reliable, and valid record of recovery from neurological deficits after a stroke. Stroke scales are based on information from the neurological examination and include measures of mentation, motor function, and language. Of available instruments, the National Institutes of Health Stroke Scale and the Canadian Neurological Scale are the best validated. Advantages of these instruments include brevity, reliability, and the fact that they can be administered by physicians, nurses, or therapists. A major limitation is that both rely on interval scales that are fairly insensitive to detecting changes. Use of a summation score can be misleading, since it combines several factors that may or may not be related.

Global Disability Measure

A global measure of disability can be used to measure stroke severity and to document recovery of function. The Rankin Scale (see Attachment 3) is the most commonly used global scale and provides a simple broad-based estimate of the amount of dependency resulting from stroke. It measures overall independence and allows comparisons to evaluate recovery over time. A limitation is that it measures only general domains of disability and lacks details to detect change.

Measures of Disability in Basic Activities of Daily Living

Measures of disability in basic ADL are used to determine the impact of impairments, establish therapeutic goals, and monitor progress in rehabilitation. They reflect both the impact of neurological impairments and the ability to compensate for losses. They focus on actual task accomplishment rather than on the theoretic ability to perform a task.

Most basic ADL scales measure multiple activities, including dressing, feeding, bathing, toileting, and mobility tasks. Some also include measures of cognition, communication, and social behavior. The information is obtained by observing performance. The Barthel Index and the Functional Independence Measure (FIM) (see Attachment 4) have been tested extensively in rehabilitation for reliability, validity, and sensitivity, and are by far the most commonly used measures. ADL measures have limitations because they are not sensitive to change in patients with high levels of functional disability (producing a *ceiling* effect); may fail to detect improvements in specific self-care activities (such as different aspects of dressing); and, by focusing on task performance, do not identify the effects of specific impairments or diseases. Also, use of summation scores can be misleading because they combine functions in different areas that are not necessarily associated.

Mental Status Assessment

Because cognitive deficits often are missed or their severity underestimated on routine neurological examinations, use of a simple, well-validated screening test can help to probe specific spheres of mental function in patients with global deficits. The Mini-Mental Status Examination (MMSE) and the Neurobehavioral Cognition Status Examination (NCSE) (see Attachment 5) are recommended. The MMSE has been used in a wide variety of populations. It has well-demonstrated validity and reliability and is brief. However, it has the disadvantage of being heavily language dependent. Therefore, it is likely to misclassify patients with aphasia. The NCSE samples a broad range of mental functions and has well-demonstrated validity, although it has not been tested for reliability in stroke.

Measures of Motor Function and Balance

The recommended instruments for measuring motor function (see Attachment 6) have been well characterized and are useful for capturing changes at the impairment level.

The Berg Balance Assessment (see Attachment 7) has well-demonstrated reliability, validity, and sensitivity to change in stroke patients.

Measures of Mobility

Physical performance measures provide insights into a patient's ability to perform basic mobility functions. They may be used for screening to determine the need for treatment, for measuring responses to treatment, and for discharge planning. The Rivermead Mobility Index (see Attachment 8) is recommended because it has been tested and used in stroke patients and is simple and reliable. Timed functional movements (e.g., time to walk 10 meters or the distance that can be walked in 6 minutes) should also be considered (Brandstater, de Bruin, Gowland, et al., 1983; Butland, Pang, Gross, et al., 1982; Lipkin, Scriven, Crake, et al., 1986; Wade and Hewer, 1987a; Wolfson, Whipple, Amerman, et al., 1990). Several instruments currently employed in geriatric screening and assessment, such as Tinetti Mobility Skills, Reuben Physical Performance, and Duke Mobility Skills, are promising but have not been evaluated in stroke populations.

Assessment of Speech and Language Function

The recommended instruments for the assessment of speech and language function (see Attachment 9) are well normed and constructed and are in wide use. These tests provide comprehensive information on speech and language disorders. They also provide a baseline against which to measure progress. Although they describe a profile of a patient's language disorder, they do not necessarily reflect measurement of functional abilities, as does the Communicative Abilities in Daily Living Test (Holland, 1980). The Functional Communication Profile (Sarno, 1969) is a rehabilitation-oriented rating scale.

Depression Scales

The instruments in Attachment 10 can be helpful in screening for depression and in monitoring responses to therapy. The instruments included are those which have been best validated in patients with stroke. Standard instruments supplement, but do not replace, the clinical interview in the diagnosis of depression.

Measures of Complex or Instrumental Activities in Daily Living

A return to independent living requires not only the ability to perform basic activities of daily living, but also the ability to carry out more complex activities (instrumental ADL) such as shopping, meal preparation, use of the telephone, driving a car, use of public transportation, money management, and desired leisure activities. The recommended instruments (see Attachment 11) are designed to measure performance of a wide range of activities in the person's living environment. Their use permits systematic monitoring of progress after the return home and provides useful measures of responses to continued outpatient or home rehabilitation.

The skills required by these complex activities are often taught during rehabilitation. Caution must be exercised, however, in extrapolating from performance in a highly supportive rehabilitation setting to the home. Structural features of the home environment, motivation, and the availability of support may each have important effects. Valid temporal comparisons must take account of these and other contextual factors.

Family Assessment Device

For assessing family functioning, a useful standardized instrument is the Family Assessment Device (FAD) (see Attachment 12). The FAD has demonstrated reliability and predictive validity (Byles, Bryne, Boyle, et al., 1988) and has been used frequently with families of stroke survivors. It contains 60 items that assess family problem solving, roles, communication, affective responsiveness, affective involvement, behavior control, and general functioning. Scores can be used to identify families that may benefit from further clinical evaluation, counseling, or education. A recent review concluded that another instrument, the DSM-IIIR Global Assessment of Functioning (GAF) Scale, is also useful in assessing the social functioning of family members (Goldman, Skodol, and Lave, 1992). This assessment device is also found in the DSM-IV™ published in 1994 (fourth edition) by the American Psychiatric Association.

Assessment of the Quality of Life

Quality of life includes the ability to engage in life's activities, the satisfaction derived from them, and overall perceptions of health status and well-being. The person's wishes and expectations, limitations in achieving these, and value system are all important factors.

Controversy continues over the ability to define quality of life, let alone measure it reliably. Nonetheless, the concept is sufficiently important and the state of the art of measurement sufficiently advanced to warrant inclusion of selected instruments as a complement to measures of IADL (in monitoring progress after a return to a community residence).

Many different measures of health status or quality of life have been developed, but only a few have been adequately validated. The recommended measures (see Attachment 13) assess a broad range of health dimensions and have been widely used. Both are generic and not specific to stroke patients. The Medical Outcomes Study 36-Item Short-Form Survey (SF-36) has the particular advantages of being brief and capable of being administered by telephone, administered in a face-to-face interview, or self-completed. Its major limitation in stroke patients is a *floor* effect which suggests that disability (ADL) measures should be added to adequately document severe disabilities. The Sickness Impact Profile (SIP) is more comprehensive and includes a broad range of items that mitigate *floor* or *ceiling* effects. Limitations are that its 136 items may take the patient 30 minutes or more to complete, and that health perception items are not included. Neither the SF-36 nor the SIP has well-documented sensitivity to detect change in stroke patients.

4 Rehabilitation During Acute Care for Stroke

Introduction

Stroke rehabilitation begins during the acute hospitalization as soon as the diagnosis of stroke is established and life-threatening problems are under control. Highest priorities are to prevent recurrent stroke, prevent complications, ensure proper management of general health functions, mobilize the patient, and encourage resumption of self-care activities as soon as medically feasible. Emotional support for patient and family during this stressful period and education in the effects of stroke and the objectives of treatment are also extremely important.

This chapter addresses:

- Benefits of acute care on dedicated stroke units.
- Clinical evaluation during acute care.
- Preventing recurrent strokes.
- Managing complications and health functions.
- Early mobilization and resumption of self-care activities.
- Needs for patient and family support and education.
- Discharge planning.

The chapter does not discuss the diagnosis or management of acute stroke; the reader is referred to up-to-date reviews of these subjects in the American Heart Association's statement on *Management of Patients with Acute Ischemic Stroke* (Adams, Brott, Crowell, et al., 1994); the National Stroke Association's consensus statement on *Stroke: the First Six Hours* (National Stroke Association, 1993); policy-relevant recommendations for the United Kingdom in the chapter on stroke in *Health Care Needs Assessment* (Wade, 1994); and reviews by Sandercock and Willems (1992) and Marshall and Mohr (1993).

Treating the Acute Stroke With Coordinated Interdisciplinary Care

Recommendation: Whenever possible, patients with acute strokes should receive coordinated diagnostic, acute management, preventive, and rehabilitative services. (Research evidence=A; expert opinion=consensus.)

Acute care hospitals vary widely in the expertise of staff in treating stroke and in the availability of rehabilitation services. Some hospitals have acute stroke units or well-staffed neurology or rehabilitation departments and can bring a full range of skills to the bedside of the patient with an acute stroke. Other hospitals have more limited capabilities or need to rely on consultants from other local hospitals.

At a minimum, the attending physician should ensure that physicians and rehabilitation specialists with expertise in stroke are closely involved in the patient's care. Serious consideration should be given to transferring the patient to a hospital with a stroke unit, if one exists in reasonable proximity and services in the admitting hospital are limited.

Acute stroke units are organized to provide coordinated services to patients with strokes and are staffed with specifically trained physicians, nurses, and rehabilitation therapists. Some evidence supports the benefits of treatment on such units (see Table 7). A meta-analysis of controlled trials found reduced mortality for up to a year after stroke in patients treated with comprehensive, coordinated rehabilitation services (Langhorne, Williams, Gilchrist, et al., 1993). Most studies also indicate improved functional outcomes, although differences in the outcome measures used make it difficult to combine results (Langhorne, Williams, Gilchrist, et al., 1993). A recent controlled trial not included in these meta-analyses found that the benefits of stroke units extended to people 75 years of age or over, and were greatest in those with strokes of intermediate severity (Kalra, Dale, and Crome, 1993).

Studies of the use of stroke teams to supplement care on general medical wards have yielded less conclusive results (Feldman, Lee, Unterecker, et al., 1962; Wood-Dauphinee, Shapiro, Bass, et al., 1984) (see Table 7).

The reasons for the favorable effects of stroke units are not known. Possibilities include better training and greater dedication of professional staff, the coordinated approach to patient care, greater success in preventing complications due to earlier mobilization of the patient and more attention to preventive measures, and emphasis on patient and family education and involvement in care.

Clinical Evaluation During Acute Care

Recommendation: The evaluation of patients with acute strokes should include initial and followup assessments of medical and neurological problems, functional health patterns, complications, and social and environmental factors that may influence discharge decisions. Information in each of these areas should be fully documented in the medical record. (Research evidence=NA; expert opinion=strong consensus.)

The objectives of clinical evaluation are to verify the diagnosis of stroke; document its etiology, pathology, and neurobehavioral manifestations; and assess any comorbid conditions or abnormalities of functional health patterns that may affect clinical management. Types of

Table 7. Evidence on the effectiveness of stroke units and stroke teams

Author Year Country	Purpose Study design Duration of deficits Number of subjects	Outcome measures Maximum followup	Conclusions/ comments
Kalra, Dale, and Crome (1993) United Kingdom	Compare SU to GMW care RCT stratified by risk score Acute deficits N=152	Mortality Discharged home LOS ADL (Barthel) F/U until hospital discharge	Mortality benefits in SU only for poor-risk group. LOS shorter in SU for intermediate- and poor-risk groups. Improved ADL in SU only for intermediate-risk group.
Indredavik, Bakke, Solberg, et al. (1991) Norway	Compare SU to GMW care RCT Acute deficits N=220	Discharged home Mortality ADL (Barthel) Neurological score F/U until 1 year	Discharge home, ADL score and neurological score favor SU at 6 weeks and 1 year. Mortality favors SU at 6 weeks.
Strand, Asplund, Eriksson, et al. (1985) Sweden	Compare nonintensive stroke unit to GMW care Non-RCT (bed availability on SU) Acute deficits N=293	Discharged home Mortality ADL F/U until 1 year	Percent discharged home and ADL at 1 year favor SU. Non-RCT design raises questions about selection bias.
Stevens, Ambler, and Warren (1984) United Kingdom	Compare nonacute stroke rehab ward (SRW) to GMW care RCT Acute deficits N=228	Mortality Discharged home ADL F/U until 1 year	Nonsignificant differences favor SRW.
Wood-Dauphinee, Shapiro, Bass, et al. (1984) Canada	Compare stroke team care to traditional care at medical unit RCT Acute deficits N=126	Mortality Motor function ADL (Barthel) F/U until 5 weeks	No significant differences in outcomes.

See notes at end of table.

Table 7. Evidence on the effectiveness of stroke units and stroke teams (continued)

Author Year Country	Purpose Study design Duration of deficits Number of subjects	Outcome measures Maximum followup	Conclusions/ comments
Garraway, Akhtar, Prescott, et al. (1980) Garraway, Akhtar, Hockey, et al. (1980) Garraway, Akhtar, Smith, et al. (1981) Smith, Garraway, Smith, et al. (1982) United Kingdom	Compare SU to GMW care RCT Acute deficits N=312	Mortality ADL F/U at discharge and 1 year	Benefits of SU noted at discharge were not sustained at 1 year. SU patients received earlier PT and OT and more OT.
Feldman, Lee, Unterecker, et al. (1962) United States	Compare inpatient care by PM&R rehabilitation staff to GMW care RCT Acute deficits N=82	Physical impairment ADL Location after discharge F/U until 1 year	No significant differences in outcomes.

Note: ADL = activities of daily living. F/U = followup. GMW = general medical ward. LOS = length of stay. OT = occupational therapy. PM&R = physical medicine and rehabilitation. PT = physical therapy. RCT = randomized controlled trial. SU = stroke unit.

information to be obtained are listed in Table 8. This information is essential in guiding treatment decisions during the acute care period. Followup examinations document responses to treatment, the evolution of neurological deficits, and any complications that may occur.

The use of simple standardized instruments facilitates systematic and reliable documentation of the patient's state of consciousness, neurological impairments, and global disability on admission and at intervals during the acute care period. Even though the clinical neurological examination addresses each of these factors, they are often incompletely or inconsistently recorded. The Glasgow Coma Scale (see Attachment 1)

Table 8. Clinical evaluation during the acute hospitalization

General clinical assessment: history, neurological and medical examinations, and selected laboratory tests
■ Functional and clinical status prior to stroke. ■ Stroke etiology and location. ■ Type(s), severity, and trajectories of neurological deficits. ■ Type(s) and severity of comorbid diseases. ■ Complications experienced during acute hospitalization. ■ Functional health patterns: nutrition and hydration, ability to swallow, bowel and bladder continence, skin integrity, activity tolerance, sleep patterns.
Social and environmental factors for discharge planning
■ Previous living situation and family support. ■ Ethnicity/language. ■ Adjustment of patient and family to illness. ■ Patient and family preferences. ■ Characteristics of potential postdischarge environments.
Standardized instruments (numbers in parentheses refer to attachment tables in this guideline)
■ Level of consciousness (1). ■ Stroke deficit scale (2). ■ Global disability scale (3).

assesses changes in levels of consciousness as manifested by eye opening, motor responses, and verbal responses to voice commands or painful stimuli. A stroke deficit scale permits systematic documentation of changes in neurological deficits in motor functions, mentation, and language (see Attachment 2). A global measure of disability such as the Rankin Scale (see Attachment 3), while relatively insensitive to change, provides a simple measure of the overall level of disability.

Discharge planning requires close involvement of the patient and family. It needs to explore social and environmental factors and preferences that will influence rehabilitation decisions, the choice of community residence, and postdischarge medical services.

Preventing Recurrent Strokes

Recommendation: Cause-specific measures to prevent recurrent stroke should be considered and implemented in all patients. (Research evidence=A; expert opinion=strong consensus.)

Patients who have had a stroke are at substantial risk of a recurrence (7 to 10 percent, per year). The choice of therapy depends on the etiology of the stroke. Surgical treatment of cerebral aneurysms after subarachnoid hemorrhage is effective in reducing recurrences in selected cases. Carotid endarterectomy should be considered in patients with minor acute ischemic stroke or transient ischemic attack, if the ipsilateral carotid artery is 70 to

99 percent obstructed. Evidence that the procedure can reduce recurrences under these circumstances is convincing, if the patient is not at major surgical risk (European Carotid Surgery Trialists Collaborative Group [ECSTCG], 1991; Mayberg, Wilson, Yatsu, et al., 1991; North American Symptomatic Carotid Endarterectomy Trial [NASCET] Collaborators, 1991). A recent clinical advisory bulletin from the National Institute of Neurological Disorders and Stroke (1994) announced the results of a clinical trial assessing carotid endarterectomy (CE) for patients with asymptomatic internal carotid artery stenosis. The trial demonstrated that CE may reduce the 5-year risk of stroke by 55 percent in patients with more than 60 percent stenosis of the carotid artery. The effectiveness of CE in lesser degrees of carotid stenosis is not known.

Anticoagulation with warfarin has been shown to reduce future cardioembolic events and/or mortality in patients with nonvalvular atrial fibrillation in five randomized clinical trials (Boston Area Anticoagulation Trial for Atrial Fibrillation, 1990; Connolly, Laupacis, Gent, et al., 1991; Ezekowitz, Bridgers, James, et al., 1992; Peterson, Boysen, Godtfredsen, et al., 1989; Stroke Prevention in Atrial Fibrillation Investigators, 1991). To achieve an acceptable benefit-to-risk ratio, clinicians should carefully monitor coagulation based on the International Normalized Ratio (INR), aiming for a ratio between 2 and 3 (Laupacis, Albers, Dunn, et al., 1992).

Antiplatelet drugs such as aspirin and ticlopidine have been shown to reduce stroke risk in patients with TIA or minor stroke (Antiplatelet Trialists Collaboration, 1988; Triclopidine Aspirin Stroke Study Group, [Bellavance], 1993). In postmyocardial infarction patients, warfarin is effective but has reported high complication rates. Aspirin should be used first for persons with TIA or minor stroke. Patients who fail aspirin, who are aspirin intolerant, or who have had a major stroke are reasonable candidates for ticlopidine (Matchar, McCrory, Barnett, et al., 1994).

Heparin is widely used for the treatment of cardiovascular abnormalities and progressive ischemic stroke (Marsh, Adams, Biller, et al., 1989) despite lack of evidence of its benefits (Adams, Brott, Crowell, et al., 1994; Jonas, 1988).

Patient education should emphasize controlling the modifiable risk factors for stroke (see Chapter 2), such as hypertension and smoking.

Preventing Venous Thromboembolism

Recommendation: Measures to prevent deep vein thrombosis (DVT) should be implemented soon after admission and continued until the patient is no longer at high risk due to immobility. (Research evidence=A; expert opinion=strong consensus.)

All stroke patients should be evaluated for the possible presence of DVT. Deep vein thrombosis is an important cause of pulmonary embolism, morbidity, and mortality after stroke. As many as 10 percent of deaths from stroke have been attributed to pulmonary embolism (Bounds, Wiebers, Whisnant, et al., 1981; Silver, Norris, Lewis, et al., 1984). The risk of DVT and thromboembolism is increased by the paralysis of a limb and resulting immobility (Landi, D'Angelo, Boccardi, et al., 1992; Warlow, Ogston, and Douglas, 1976), and thromboembolism has been reported to occur in as many as 47 percent of untreated patients (Clagett, Anderson, and Levine, 1992). Pooled results from randomized trials have shown a 45 percent risk reduction with prophylaxis using low-dose heparin (LDH) and a 79 percent reduction with low-molecular-weight (LMW) heparin (Brandstater, Roth, and Siebens, 1992; Clagett, Anderson, and Levine, 1992; Sandercock and Willems, 1992). The Clagett article concluded that LDH and LMW heparin are preferred treatments and that warfarin, intermittent pneumatic compression, and elastic stockings are also effective. Management of the stroke patient should include early mobilization, use of elastic stockings, and, in the absence of contraindications, prophylaxis with one of the preferred agents.

Managing Complications

Managing Dysphagia and Preventing Aspiration

Recommendation: The patient's ability to swallow should be assessed soon after admission and before oral intake of fluids or food is begun. Training in techniques to facilitate swallowing should be implemented as soon as possible in patients with a swallowing disorder. (Research evidence=C; expert opinion=strong consensus.)

Dysphagia (impaired swallowing) occurs frequently in stroke patients and may result in aspiration and pneumonia if not diagnosed and appropriately managed (Horner, Massey, Riski, et al., 1988; Palmer and DeChase, 1991). Aspiration is silent in as many as 40 percent of patients who aspirate. Fortunately, spontaneous improvement is frequent.

The clinical assessment of dysphagia is discussed in Chapter 3. The goals of management are to prevent aspiration, prevent dehydration and malnutrition from inadequate oral intake, and restore the patient's ability to chew and swallow safely. Compensatory treatments involve changes in posture and positioning for swallowing, learning of new swallowing maneuvers, changes in the texture of foods (e.g., thickening liquids and using pureed or semisolid foods), decreasing bolus size, and administering food by syringe. Patients who do not regain the ability to swallow safely will require parenteral or tube feeding. If long-term tube feeding is required, a gastrostomy is usually preferable to a nasogastric tube (Emick-Herring and Wood, 1990).

Evidence supporting the effectiveness of treatment is from observational studies. A carefully performed large case series found that 89 percent of patients were able to resume oral feeding and none developed aspiration pneumonia after a compensatory feeding program

(Horner, Massey, Riski, et al., 1988). Controlled trials will be needed to compare the effectiveness of different treatment regimens.

Maintaining Skin Integrity

Recommendation: Measures to maintain skin integrity should be initiated during acute care and continued throughout rehabilitation. (Research evidence=C; expert opinion=strong consensus.)

The National Survey of Stroke found that 14.5 percent of stroke patients develop pressure sores (Roth, 1991). Patients who are comatose, severely paralyzed, obese, or incontinent of bladder or bowel, or who have muscle spasticity are at unusually high risk. Steps to maintain skin integrity include:

- Systematic daily inspection of the skin to detect areas of incipient breakdown, paying particular attention to areas over bony prominences.
- Gentle routine skin cleansing.
- Protection from exposure to moisture (e.g., urine, perspiration).
- Avoidance of skin injury due to friction or excessive pressure through use of proper positioning, turning, and transferring techniques; and by judicious use of barrier sprays, lubricants, special mattresses, and protective dressings and padding.
- Careful attention to the maintenance of adequate hydration and nutrition.
- Efforts to improve the patient's mobility.

If the patient remains incontinent despite efforts to treat the specific cause, condom drainage in men and diapering products in men and women can help minimize the contact of urine with the skin. Prior to discharge from acute care, the patient and family need to be fully instructed in the techniques of skin care and prevention of skin breakdown. For a full discussion of skin breakdown, with recommendations for prevention and treatment of Stage I pressure ulcers, refer to the AHCPR-sponsored guideline, *Pressure Ulcers in Adults: Prediction and Prevention* (Panel for the Prediction and Prevention of Pressure Ulcers in Adults, 1992).

Preventing Falls

Recommendation: The patient's risk of falling should be assessed at the time of admission and updated regularly during recovery. Methods to prevent falls depend on the type(s) and severity of the patient's disabilities. (Research evidence=C; expert opinion=strong consensus.)

Falls are the most frequent cause of injury in patients hospitalized with strokes. Hip fracture is a common complication (Poplingher and Pillar, 1985). The risk of falls is increased by sensorimotor deficits that lead to problems with mobility, balance, or coordination; and by confusion, perceptual deficits, visual impairments, and problems with communication that interfere with a patient's ability to ask for assistance or make needs known. Acute illnesses, generalized weakness, and drug side effects compound risks due to neurological deficits. Patients with visual neglect and those who are slow in performing tasks are at unusually high risk of multiple accidents (Diller and Weinberg, 1970) and of running into obstacles (Webster, Rapport, Godlewski, et al., 1994). Behavioral impulsivity, older age, a history of previous falls, and multiple transfers increase the risk of falls in patients with right hemisphere strokes (Rapport, Webster, Fleming, et al., 1993).

Assessment should address the patient's risk factors and also potential hazards in the hospital environment (e.g., the surface of floors, lighting, and placement of and access to toilet facilities). The nursing staff usually has primary responsibility for assessment and for implementing preventive measures, but all clinicians should participate in fall prevention. A risk reduction program includes careful supervision of high-risk patients, toileting at regular intervals, supervised transfer and ambulation, nurse call systems suited to a patient's abilities, hospital-wide fall prevention programs, and—extremely important—adequate patient and family education.

Managing Bladder Function

Recommendation: In cases where a catheter is inserted during the acute phase, the catheter should be removed as soon as possible. Chronic use of indwelling catheters should be limited to patients in whom incontinence or urinary retention cannot be otherwise treated. (Research evidence=C; expert opinion=strong consensus.)

Problems with bladder control and incontinence are common after stroke, but they resolve spontaneously in the large majority of patients (Brocklehurst, Andrews, Richards, et al., 1985). Causes include neurological deficits that lead to bladder hypertonicity, bladder hypotonicity with overflow incontinence, or cognitive or communication deficits with the resultant inability to recognize the need to void or to make the need known (Gelber, Good, Laven, et al., 1993). Persistent incontinence confers a poor long-term prognosis for functional recovery (Jongbloed, 1986; Reding, Winter, Hochrein, et al., 1987).

Use of an indwelling catheter should be limited to patients with incontinence due to urinary retention that cannot be otherwise treated, severely impaired patients with skin breakdown in whom frequent bed or clothing changes would be difficult or painful, and patients in whom incontinence interferes with monitoring of fluid and electrolyte balance. Chronic use of indwelling catheters increases the risk of bacteriuria and urinary tract infection (Bjork, Pelletier, and Tight, 1984; Sabanthan, Castleden, and Mitchell, 1985; Warren, Tenney, Hoopes, et al., 1982) and should be avoided (Sedrat and Hecht, 1993). Urinary retention can be safely managed with clean intermittent catheterization (Bennett and

Diokno, 1984; Maynard and Diokno, 1984; Webb, Lawson, and Neal, 1990). Whether an indwelling or intermittent straight catheter is used, good catheter care is the best way to prevent urinary infection. Bacteriuria can be identified by urine cultures, but treatment with antibiotics should generally be reserved for patients with symptomatic urinary tract infections.

For further discussion of the management of urinary incontinence, see the AHCPR-sponsored guideline, *Urinary Incontinence in Adults* (Urinary Incontinence Guideline Panel, 1992).

Preventing or Controlling Seizures

Recommendation: Patients who have had seizures after stroke should be given anticonvulsant medication to prevent recurrent seizures. (Research evidence=NA; expert opinion=consensus.)

Seizures are a potential complication of stroke and, if not controlled, can be potentially life threatening. Seizures can occur at the time of the acute stroke, during the first few days, or several months after the event. No study has specifically tested the usefulness of anticonvulsant medications in preventing or controlling seizures following stroke. Drugs that have been proven to be of value in preventing seizures of other causes, however, are recommended for patients who have had one or more seizures following stroke. The routine prophylactic administration of anticonvulsants to stroke survivors who have not had seizures should be avoided.

Early Mobilization and Return to Self Care

Recommendation: The patient with an acute stroke should be mobilized as soon after admission as is medically feasible. (Research evidence=C; expert opinion=strong consensus.)

Recommendation: The patient should be encouraged to perform self-care activities as soon as medically feasible and, if necessary, should be offered compensatory training to overcome disabilities. (Research evidence=NA; expert opinion=strong consensus.)

Early mobilization helps prevent DVT, skin breakdown, contracture formation, constipation, and pneumonia. It has positive psychological effects on both the patient and the family. Direct evidence of benefit is provided by controlled studies that have shown better orthostatic tolerance and earlier improvement of ADL performance (Asberg, 1989); earlier ambulation (Hayes and Carroll, 1986); and earlier return of mental, motor, and ADL performance (Hamrin, 1982a and 1982b) (see Table 9). Benefits in these studies were transient, however, and bias cannot be excluded since none used randomization to assign subjects to treatment or control groups.

Table 9. Evidence on the benefits of early mobilization of the stroke patient

Author Year Country	Purpose Study design Duration of deficits Number of subjects	Outcome measures Maximum followup	Conclusions/ comments
Asberg (1989) Sweden	Test benefits of early activation of the patient after an acute stroke Non-RCT (two wards admitted on alternate days) Acute deficits N=63	Orthostatic tolerance ADL (Katz) F/U until 3 months	Early activation improved orthostatic tolerance and led to transient ADL benefit. Not clear whether ADL effects were due to early activation or to increased nurse contact.
Hayes and Carroll (1986) United States	Test benefits of early rehabilitation Non-RCT Acute deficits N=30	Ambulatory ability ADL F/U until discharge	Nonsignificant results to favor early intervention. No significant differences in outcomes.
Hamrin (1982a and 1982b) Sweden	Test early activation in daily nursing care Non-RCT Acute deficits N=112	Activity index Mortality F/U until 3 months	No significant differences at discharge or 3 months.

Note: ADL = activities of daily living. F/U = followup. RCT = randomized controlled trial.

Indirect evidence of the benefits of early mobilization and rehabilitation therapy is suggested by the superiority of acute care stroke units in reducing mortality and improving functional outcomes. Early mobilization and early implementation of therapy are intrinsic components of care on stroke units and may have contributed to improved outcomes.

Mobilization is recommended as soon as the patient's medical and neurological condition permits and, if possible, within 24 to 48 hours of admission. Mobilization will need to be delayed or approached with caution in patients with coma, severe obtundation, progressing neurological signs or symptoms, subarachnoid or intracerebral hemorrhage, severe or persistent orthostatic hypotension, and acute myocardial infarction.

The rate and extent of mobilization depend on the patient's condition. Frequent position changes in bed and daily passive and active range of motion exercises of limbs are part of care from the time of admission. Proper positioning helps reduce the risk of aspiration, skin breakdown, joint contractures, and injury to joints in involved limbs. Important considerations include using a pullsheet to pull a patient up in bed rather than lifting under the arms, ensuring maintenance of therapeutic positions and the support of limbs in anatomically normal positions, and adequate support in bed. Range of motion exercises of joints in involved limbs reduce the risk of contracture and DVT.

Assessment of mobility begins with evaluating the patient's ability to turn from side to side and move up and sit up in bed, and then progresses to examining the ability to sit on the edge of the bed. Assistance and guarding are required when sitting is begun to protect both the patient and provider. The possibility of orthostatic hypotension needs to be carefully monitored. Mobilization progresses to patient transfers to a chair, commode, sofa, or wheelchair (and sitting on these); and finally coming to a standing position, bearing weight, and walking. Decisions on appropriate seating depend on sitting balance, endurance, and the need for pressure reduction. Safety, comfort, and maximizing mobility and independence are each important considerations. Transfer techniques should be taught by rehabilitation professionals who are expert in them. These techniques need to be used consistently by all who transfer the patient.

Self-care activities such as eating, grooming, toileting, and dressing should also be encouraged as soon as possible. Active participation in self care helps the patient resume control and increase strength, endurance, and awareness of the environment. Compensatory training can facilitate progress by teaching adaptive techniques to overcome disabilities. Mental activity is as important as physical activities, and efforts to encourage communication, problem solving, and social activity are very much part of the acute care process in suitable patients.

Patient and Family Support and Education During the Acute Hospitalization

Recommendation: Patients who survive the acute stroke, and their families, should be thoroughly instructed in the effects and prognosis of the stroke, potential complications, and the needs and rationales for treatments. (Research evidence=NA; expert opinion=consensus.)

Stroke is a catastrophic event for the patient and family. Survivors have to confront resulting disabilities and the pervasive effects a stroke may have on their lives. Families, in turn, have to learn to provide support and adjust to altered relationships with a family member who has disabilities.

Important goals are to provide support for the patient and family during this time of need and to ensure that they gain a realistic understanding of the consequences of stroke and the objectives and methods of various treatments. Since the anxiety and stress associated with an acute stroke often interfere with the ability of the patient and family to comprehend the full meaning of the event or its treatment, understanding rather than mere explanation must be a goal of education.

Planning for Discharge From Acute Care

Recommendation: Discharge planning should begin at the time of admission. Goals are to determine the need for rehabilitation, arrange the best possible living environment, and assure continuity of care after discharge. (Research evidence=NA; expert opinion=strong consensus.)

Effective discharge planning will contribute to better patient outcomes and at the same time help to improve the efficiency and cost effectiveness of hospital care. The family and patient need to be intimately involved in the process of exploring needs and expectations for future medical and rehabilitative services and potential living options. Patient and family preferences and the availability of support by family or involved others will be important determinants of the decisions that are made. While final arrangements will depend primarily on the patient's clinical course, early attention to these issues will greatly facilitate timely discharges.

Health professionals who are responsible for the patient's care during the acute hospitalization are also responsible for ensuring continuity of services following discharge. An important part of this responsibility is identifying patients who are candidates for a structured rehabilitation program. Decisions about referral to further rehabilitation are the subject of Chapter 5. Screening procedures should be implemented as soon as the patient's medical and neurological status permits.

5 Screening for Rehabilitation and Choice of a Setting

Introduction

Many people who have had a stroke require assistance in adjusting to disabilities after stroke, and some are candidates for a rehabilitation program. The need for rehabilitation should be considered as soon as the patient's medical and neurological status has stabilized.

Figure 4 summarizes the process of reaching a rehabilitation decision. This decision is based primarily on information gathered during a screening examination. The overall goal is to achieve the best possible match between the needs of the patient and the capabilities of rehabilitation programs available in a community. Limited options for rehabilitation in some communities, particularly in rural areas, may restrict choices.

Recommendations in this chapter are focused on the initial rehabilitation decision following an acute hospitalization for a stroke. However, they also apply to changes in the rehabilitation setting or the level of care during later stages of recovery. The recommendations are based almost entirely on the judgments of experts in rehabilitation. Although the available evidence (see Table 10) suggests that rehabilitation is beneficial to some patients, no study has clearly demonstrated the superiority of one type of program or rehabilitation setting over another or specifically identified the characteristics of patients most likely to benefit.

Screening for Rehabilitation

Recommendation: Screening for possible admission to a rehabilitation program should be performed as soon as the patient's neurological and medical condition permits. The individual(s) performing the screening examination should be experienced in stroke rehabilitation and preferably should have no direct financial interest in the referral decision. All screening information should be summarized in the acute medical record and provided to the rehabilitation setting at the time of referral. (Research evidence=NA; expert opinion=strong consensus.)

The purpose of the screening examination is to identify patients who need rehabilitation and to select the best possible rehabilitation setting. Patients will not require a complete screening examination if they are clearly not candidates for rehabilitation. This is because they have either recovered completely or they are too disabled by paralyses, cognitive problems, or comorbid conditions to participate gainfully.

The screening examination should be sensitive to the concerns of patient and family and to their needs for understanding, caring, and

Figure 4. Framework for rehabilitation decisions

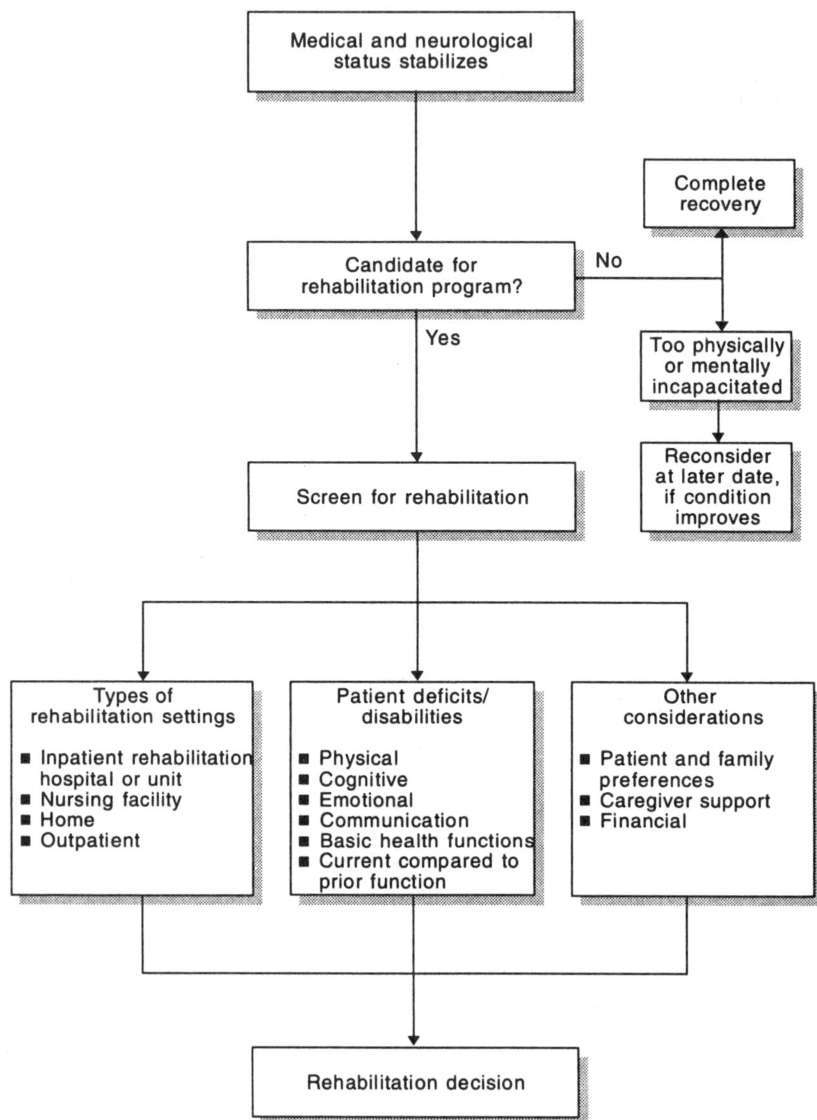

Table 10. Evidence on the effectiveness of rehabilitation in different types of settings

Author Year Country	Purpose Study design Duration of deficits Number of subjects	Outcome measures Maximum followup	Conclusions/ comments
Young and Forster (1991 and 1992) United Kingdom	Compare day hospital with home physiotherapy RCT stratified by time since onset and disability level Acute deficits N=125	Functional ambulation ADL (Barthel) Motor Club Assessment Frenchay Activities Index Nottingham Health Profile General Health Questionnaire F/U until 6 months	Home physiotherapy significantly more effective and resource efficient.
Wade, Collen, Robb, et al. (1992) United Kingdom	Test whether outpatient PT improves mobility in chronic stroke patients RCT with crossover Chronic deficits N=94	Motricity Index Functional Ambulation Categories Rivermead Motor Assessment Frenchay Activities Index Gait speed Rivermead Mobility Index Nottingham Extended ADL Index Hospital Anxiety and Depression Scale Nine-hole peg test	Outpatient PT increases gait speed in chronic stroke patients, but benefits decline after therapy stopped.
Wade, Langton-Hewer, Skilbeck, et al. (1985) United Kingdom	Examine value of home-care services for stroke patients Non-RCT Acute deficits N=857	ADL (Barthel) Frenchay Activities Index Wakefield Depression Inventory General Health Questionnaire (for caregivers) F/U until 6 months	No difference in functional recovery or stress on caregivers.

See notes at end of table.

Table 10. Evidence on the effectiveness of rehabilitation in different types of settings (continued)

Author Year Country	Purpose Study design Duration of deficits Number of subjects	Outcome measures Maximum followup	Conclusions/ comments
Sivenius, Pyorala, Heinonen, et al. (1985) Finland	Compare intensive rehab therapy (IT) to conventional rehab in an acute care hospital RCT Acute deficits N=95	Motor function ADL (Lehmann) Mortality F/U until 1 year	Motor function score better in IT group until 1 year and ADL score until 3 months. No differences in mortality. Differences in baseline function raise questions about the success of randomization.
Tucker, Davison, and Ogle (1984) New Zealand	Examine benefits of day hospital rehabilitation RCT NA N=120	ADL (Northwick Park) Zung Depression Scale F/U until 5 months	Day hospital group improved more on ADL at 6 weeks and depression score up to 5 months, but cost higher than usual care. No significant differences in outcomes.
Smith, Goldenberg, Ashburn, et al. (1981) United Kingdom	Test whether more intensive OP rehab improves outcomes RCT Acute deficits N=133	Mortality ADL F/U until 12 months	Graded response of ADL to intensity of treatment with significant differences between intense rehab and no formal treatment up to 1 year.

See notes at end of table.

support. This implies that screening should cast a relatively broad net in an effort to identify all patients who are likely to benefit from rehabilitation. Subsequent detailed assessment by the rehabilitation program can then validate the appropriateness of the referral. Also, screening must be practical in terms of the time, effort, and skills required.

Table 10. Evidence on the effectiveness of rehabilitation in different types of settings (continued)

Author Year Country	Purpose Study design Duration of deficits Number of subjects	Outcome measures Maximum followup	Conclusions/ comments
Feigenson, Gitlow, and Greenberg (1979) United States	Test whether a stroke-dedicated rehab unit in a facility achieves better outcomes than multiple diagnosis rehab units Retrospective non-RCT Acute deficits N=667	Ambulation ADL Length of stay Discharged home Mortality F/U until discharge	Functional outcomes similar despite more severe neurological deficits in stroke-only unit at the time of admission.

Note: ADL = activities of daily living. F/U = followup. NA = not available. OP = outpatient. PT = physical therapy. RCT = randomized controlled trial. Rehab = rehabilitation.

Areas of information covered by the screening examination are listed in Table 11. This examination can be completed in 1 hour or less by a well-trained rehabilitation clinician if the medical record contains a complete and current description of neurological deficits, comorbid diseases, and functional health patterns.

The patient's medical stability and the nature and extent of functional limitations are the most important determinants of the need for rehabilitation and the appropriate choice of a rehabilitation program or service. The functional status and degree of independence prior to the stroke provide reasonable upper bounds on expectations for rehabilitation.

The patient's ability to tolerate the physical activity required by rehabilitation should be carefully evaluated. Cardiopulmonary endurance and the muscle strength of uninvolved limbs must be sufficient to permit training in mobility and ADL. Major orthopedic problems such as severe arthritis may also limit rehabilitation. Evaluation of patients with compromised physical activity endurance should attempt to distinguish cardiopulmonary limitations due to deconditioning from those due to major cardiovascular or pulmonary comorbidity.

Information on social, cultural, economic, and environmental factors is best obtained through interviews with the patient and family. Expectations for rehabilitation and preferences for choice of setting should be explored, since rehabilitation is more likely to be successful if the patient and family are fully supportive. The program choice may also be influenced by the home environment—whether the structural characteristics of the home

Table 11. Screening for rehabilitation

Current clinical status ■ Neurological deficits. ■ Comorbid diseases. ■ Functional health patterns: nutrition and hydration, ability to swallow, bowel and bladder continence, skin integrity, activity tolerance, sleep patterns.
Special emphases ■ Functional status prior to stroke. ■ Current functional deficits. ■ Mental status and ability to learn. ■ Emotional status and motivation to participate in rehabilitation. ■ Functional communication. ■ Physical activity endurance.
Social and environmental factors[a] ■ Presence of spouse or significant other. ■ Previous living situation. ■ Ethnicity and native language. ■ Adjustment of patient and family to stroke. ■ Patient and family preferences for and expectations of rehabilitation. ■ Extent of support by family or involved others (relationships, number, health, availability). ■ Characteristics of potential postdischarge environments.
Standardized instruments (numbers in parentheses refer to attachment tables in this guideline) ■ Stroke deficit scale (2). ■ Measure of disability (ADL) (4). ■ Mental status screening test (5).

[a]For more information on social and environmental factors, see Table 6 in Chapter 3.

Note: ADL = activities of daily living.

permit rehabilitation to take place there or will provide a suitable residence after rehabilitation. The availability of family members or involved others to participate in rehabilitation and to provide support at home are especially important.

Standardized instruments are recommended to document levels of neurological impairments and disabilities. An updated assessment on the National Institutes of Health Stroke Scale or the Canadian Neurological Scale used during acute care (see Attachment 2) serves as a benchmark for assessing future neurological improvements. Use of a disability (ADL) scale (see Attachment 4) permits reliable documentation of the performance of basic ADL such as mobility, dressing, grooming, eating, and toileting. The Functional Independence Measure (FIM) has the advantage of including measures of cognitive function, communication, and social functioning. A mental status screening test (see Attachment 5) is useful to document cognitive deficits that may not be readily evident during routine neurological examinations.

Because of the complexity of issues involved in rehabilitation decisions, screening should be performed (whenever possible) by a medically trained person with specialized training in stroke rehabilitation and in the reliable administration of the recommended standardized instruments. To minimize the potential for bias, the screening clinician ideally should have no direct financial interest in the referral decision. Decisions based on incomplete information or on triage relying solely on information from referring physicians not trained in rehabilitation are discouraged.

Additional time and effort spent on a thorough screening examination will better serve the interests of the patient and family and will also lead to more cost-effective use of stroke rehabilitation resources.

Rehabilitation Programs and Settings

Stroke rehabilitation following discharge from acute care can be conducted in inpatient rehabilitation hospitals or rehabilitation units in acute care hospitals, nursing facilities, the patient's home, or outpatient facilities. The capabilities typical of each type of setting will be discussed.

Hospital Inpatient Rehabilitation

Programs of rehabilitation hospitals or rehabilitation units in acute care hospitals are staffed by the full range of rehabilitation professionals—nurses, physical and occupational therapists, speech-language pathologists, psychologists, social workers, recreational therapists, and physicians. A physician skilled in rehabilitation is available 24 hours a day. An interdisciplinary team drawing on these professionals provides a comprehensive rehabilitation program for each patient. Team conferences are held at least weekly to establish rehabilitation goals and develop a rehabilitation plan, assess patient progress, identify barriers or complications and revise the rehabilitation goals or plan accordingly, and develop a plan for discharge or transfer to another type of rehabilitation program (National Association of Rehabilitation Facilities, 1988).

Hospital-level rehabilitation is usually more intense and comprehensive than rehabilitation in other settings and requires greater physical and mental effort from the patient.

Rehabilitation in Nursing Facilities

Rehabilitation programs in nursing facilities vary widely in their capabilities. Traditionally, nursing homes have provided supportive care and low-level rehabilitation services. More recently, however, some nursing facilities have developed coordinated rehabilitation programs that are similar to, though usually less intense than, hospital programs. Physician coverage in nursing facilities varies.

Nursing facilities may be either hospital based or community based. Hospital-based nursing facilities are designed primarily for patients who have the potential to improve enough during 2 or 3 weeks of treatment to become suitable candidates for inpatient hospital, home, or outpatient rehabilitation. Community-based nursing facilities run the full gamut of comprehensiveness and intensity of services. Some offer comprehensive programs providing a thorough evaluation at the time of admission, medical management by a qualified rehabilitation physician, 24-hour nursing care, and interdisciplinary treatment. At the other end of the spectrum are nursing facilities with limited rehabilitation capabilities that provide physical therapy and occupational therapy for up to 1 hour a day, 5 days per week—are staffed with nurses who may or may not have special training in rehabilitation—and are usually covered by physicians with no specific training in rehabilitation.

This diversity among nursing facility programs underscores the need for referring clinicians to inform themselves about the capabilities of individual programs.

Outpatient Rehabilitation

Outpatient rehabilitation is provided by hospital outpatient departments and freestanding outpatient facilities. These facilities can provide either a comprehensive rehabilitation program or individual rehabilitation services. Intensity may range from occasional visits to three or four visits per week. Advantages of outpatient programs are the access they permit to an interdisciplinary program, the availability of rehabilitation equipment, and the opportunity for social contact and peer support while the patient lives at home. The availability of transportation is a prerequisite.

Day hospital programs are similar to outpatient programs though frequently more intense. The patient spends several hours, 3 to 5 days a week, in a typical day hospital program. Availability of transportation is a prerequisite for both outpatient and day hospital programs.

Home Rehabilitation

Home rehabilitation programs are expanding their capabilities. Most programs are designed for patients who are medically stable and require only intermittent contact with physical or occupational therapy or nursing services. However, some home health agencies provide the full scope of services including nursing, physical therapy, occupational therapy, speech therapy, medical social services and personal care services, as well as rehabilitation nursing and mental health nursing. Recently, some home rehabilitation programs have been developed that provide comprehensive services including 24-hour coverage by physicians (Portnow, Kline, Daly, et al., 1991). The usefulness and cost effectiveness of these programs have not been fully evaluated. In programs approved by Medicare, a physician and an interdisciplinary team develop the treatment plan and monitor medical stability.

Advantages of home care programs are that rehabilitation takes place in the same environment where the skills learned will be applied, and that many patients function better in a familiar environment. Disadvantages include an increased burden on caregivers, less availability of physician monitoring, absence of peer support from fellow patients, and limited availability in the home of equipment used in facility-based inpatient or outpatient rehabilitation programs. Home rehabilitation may be the only choice for patients who would be suitable for outpatient rehabilitation but lack transportation. For some patients, a combination of outpatient and home rehabilitation may be beneficial.

The Need for Accurate Program Information

Recommendation: Rehabilitation programs should maintain up-to-date information on staffing patterns, services offered, and quality indicators and outcomes and should make this information widely available to health care providers, medical facilities, and the public. Health care providers and hospitals who refer patients to rehabilitation programs should be knowledgeable about the capabilities of programs in their communities. (Research evidence=NA; expert opinion=consensus.)

Rehabilitation decisions will better serve the needs of patients if they are based on objective information on the capabilities and actual performance of rehabilitation facilities. In spite of efforts to establish standards, the capabilities of programs in each type of setting vary widely.

Freestanding rehabilitation hospitals, rehabilitation units of acute care hospitals, and nursing facility programs that have been certified by the Commission on Accreditation of Rehabilitation Facilities (CARF)[1] and the Joint Commission on Accreditation of Healthcare Organizations (JCAHO)[2] are required to meet specific structural, staffing, and program standards. However, the ability to satisfy these accreditation standards does not guarantee uniform capabilities and quality of care.

Rehabilitation hospitals or nursing facility programs that have not been certified by CARF or JCAHO, outpatient departments, and home care agencies currently lack uniform standards. Local initiatives to obtain

[1]The CARF address for correspondence is 101 North Wilmot Road, Suite 500, Tucson, AZ 85711. Telephone: (602) 748-1212.
[2]The JCAHO address for correspondence is 1 Renaissance Boulevard, Oak Brook Terrace, IL 61081. Telephone: (708) 916-5600.

information about these programs will be especially important until regional or national standards can be developed and implemented.[3]

Definitions

The recommendations in this chapter relating patient characteristics to decisions on the appropriate type of rehabilitation setting use the following definitions.

Medical Stability

Medical stability is an important consideration affecting the patient's readiness for rehabilitation and the choice of rehabilitation setting. Degrees of medical stability are defined as follows:

- **Stable.** Patient is afebrile, has stable vital signs, and has had no important changes in medical conditions, nor required changes in treatments within the preceding 48 hours. Neurological deficits are unchanged or improving. The patient can take adequate nutrition orally or an enteral route for nutrition and hydration has been established.
- **Moderately stable.** One or more medical problems has required a change in medications within the preceding 48 hours, but symptoms or clinical findings have not changed significantly. An adequate route for nutrition and hydration has not been established. Neurological deficits are unchanged or improving.
- **Unstable.** Patient has undiagnosed or inadequately treated cardiac arrhythmia, congestive heart failure, or other condition that requires the diagnostic or treatment capabilities of an acute care hospital. The condition may be life threatening, may lead to severe morbidity if not promptly treated, or will interfere with rehabilitation. Neurological deficits or state of consciousness have fluctuated within the preceding 48 hours.

Functional Disabilities

The functions considered here are mobility (e.g., getting out of bed, walking or climbing stairs, using a wheelchair) and performance of basic ADL (e.g., eating, grooming, and dressing). Levels of disability are classified as:

- **Complete independence.** Ability to perform the activity safely and within a reasonable period of time with no assistance.

---

[3]CARF has proposed a new classification scheme for rehabilitation that includes a broadened range of nursing facility programs. CARF also plans to develop accreditation for home programs.

- **Modified independence.** Activity performance requires specialized equipment or takes more than a reasonable time or requires safety precautions, but no helper is needed.
- **Supervision or setup.** Activity requires verbal encouragement or instructions or assistance with preparation (such as opening containers or applying toothpaste to a brush), but no contact assistance.
- **Minimal contact assistance.** Ability to perform 75 percent or more of the activity unassisted; physical assistance required for the remainder.
- **Moderate assistance.** Ability to perform 50 to 74 percent of the activity unassisted; physical assistance required for the remainder.
- **Maximal assistance.** Ability to perform 25 to 49 percent of the activity unassisted; physical assistance required for the remainder.
- **Total assistance.** Ability to perform less than 25 percent of the activity unassisted; physical assistance required for the remainder.

Mental Status

Mental status affects the patient's ability to learn and retain the lessons being taught during rehabilitation. Mental status includes the degree of alertness, orientation, memory, control of behavior, and problem-solving ability. Levels of impairment are classified as:

- **Normal or minimal deficit.** Patient is alert and fully oriented, performs well on simple tests of recent memory, is consistently in control of behavior and emotions, and is easily able to follow 2-step directions.
- **Moderate deficit.** Patient is intermittently confused in time or place, or recent memory is impaired but patient is able to retain simple messages after multiple repetitions, or patient makes frequent mistakes in following 2-step directions.
- **Severe deficit.** Patient is consistently disoriented in time and place, or recent memory is severely impaired, or patient is unable to follow 2-step directions.

Physical Activity Endurance

The physical demands of rehabilitation are substantial, particularly in light of the increased effort required by the presence of hemiparesis. Physical endurance is categorized by the time a person is able to engage in physically demanding activity equivalent to that required during active rehabilitation interventions:

- 3 or more hours of physical activity per day.
- 1 to 3 hours.
- Less than 1 hour.

A threshold criterion for admission to any rehabilitation program is defined as the ability to sit supported for at least 1 hour *and* at least some ability to participate actively in rehabilitation interventions.

Caregiver Support

The patient's previous living environment and the availability of family or friends to provide assistance after discharge may influence rehabilitation decisions. Assessing the adequacy of caregiver support requires a qualitative judgment by the screening clinician.

Rehabilitation Decisions

The Need for Consensus

Recommendation: To the maximum extent possible, decisions about entry into a rehabilitation program should reflect a consensus among the patient, family or involved others, physician (in collaboration with care providers), and the rehabilitation program. (Research evidence=NA; expert opinion=strong consensus.)

Rehabilitation is fundamentally a patient-centered process that also intimately involves the family (using the term "family" broadly to include other involved persons as well). This requires the full support and active participation of the patient and family. Hence, rehabilitation decisions need to be mutually acceptable to all involved parties. Patient and family education about stroke rehabilitation, its goals and procedures, available programs, and their outcomes provide important inputs. Sensitivity to language problems and to cultural differences is important. In making a recommendation about rehabilitation to the patient and family, clinicians need to explain clearly the reasons for the recommendation and listen carefully to any concerns the patient or family have that may dictate a different choice. For example, the program that is best from a clinical point of view might be unaffordable, might be located too far away for frequent family visits, or might have characteristics or sponsorship with which the family is not comfortable.

Threshold Criteria for Admission to a Rehabilitation Program

Recommendation: The most important determinants of the need for a rehabilitation program are the patient's type/types and severity/severities of impairments and functional disabilities, the ability to learn, and physical activity endurance. (Research evidence=NA; expert opinion=strong consensus.)

Threshold patient characteristics for entry into any active rehabilitation program are shown in Figure 5. Terms were defined earlier in the chapter. Threshold criteria are (1) patient is medically stable or moderately stable, (2) patient has one or more persistent disabilities, (3) patient is able to learn, and (4) patient has enough physical activity endurance to sit supported for at least 1 hour a day and to participate actively in rehabilitation (physical endurance less than this minimal level indicates that rehabilitation services at home or in a supportive living setting would be a better choice).

Patients who are too debilitated to participate in an active rehabilitation program may benefit from a brief interdisciplinary program designed to educate the family and provide "hands-on" training in the skills needed to maintain a severely disabled patient at home. Objectives of such a program are to ensure that the family has a thorough understanding of the patient's impairments, the risks they entail, and opportunities and techniques for maximizing function. This type of program can be conducted in a rehabilitation facility (hospital or nursing facility), a day program, or at home. A facility-based program makes it easier to involve multiple professional disciplines and provide access to needed equipment; a home program has the advantage of enabling the training to be adapted to the actual home environment.

Recommendation: Admission to an interdisciplinary rehabilitation program should generally be limited to patients with disabilities in two or more of the following areas of function: mobility, performance of the basic activities of daily living, bowel or bladder control, cognition, emotional functioning, pain management, swallowing, and communication. (Research evidence=NA; expert opinion=consensus.)

An isolated disability can usually be treated by services rendered by an individual rehabilitation discipline and does not require the involvement of an interdisciplinary team. Examples would be treatment of isolated motor weakness of the leg or the arm, or treatment of aphasia. The presence of cognitive, emotional, or other problems that increase the complexity of rehabilitation may require an interdisciplinary approach even though physical disabilities are mild.

The Choice of Rehabilitation Setting

For people who meet the preceding threshold criteria, the selection of setting will depend on the patient's medical stability, level of function, mental status, and physical activity endurance; the adequacy of support by family or involved others; the adequacy of the living environment; and the capabilities of rehabilitation facilities in the community. Strong contextual support often broadens the array of options. The relationships between these factors and the choice of type of rehabilitation program are shown in Figure 5.

Figure 5. Selection of setting for rehabilitation program after hospitalization for acute stroke

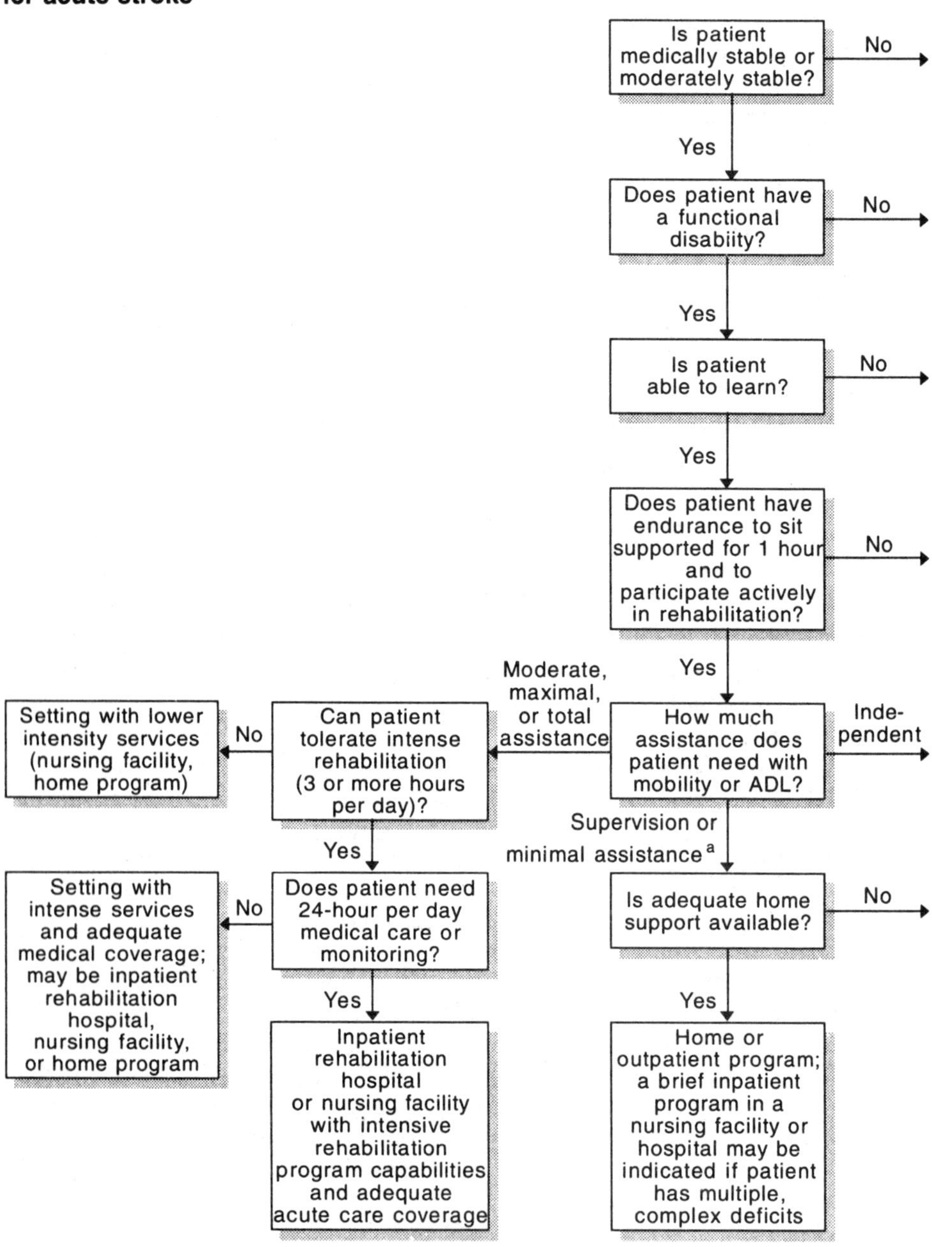

[a]Under special circumstances, some patients with multiple, complex, functional deficits may be appropriate for inpatient programs.

Note: ADL = activities of daily living. IADL = instrumental activities of daily living.

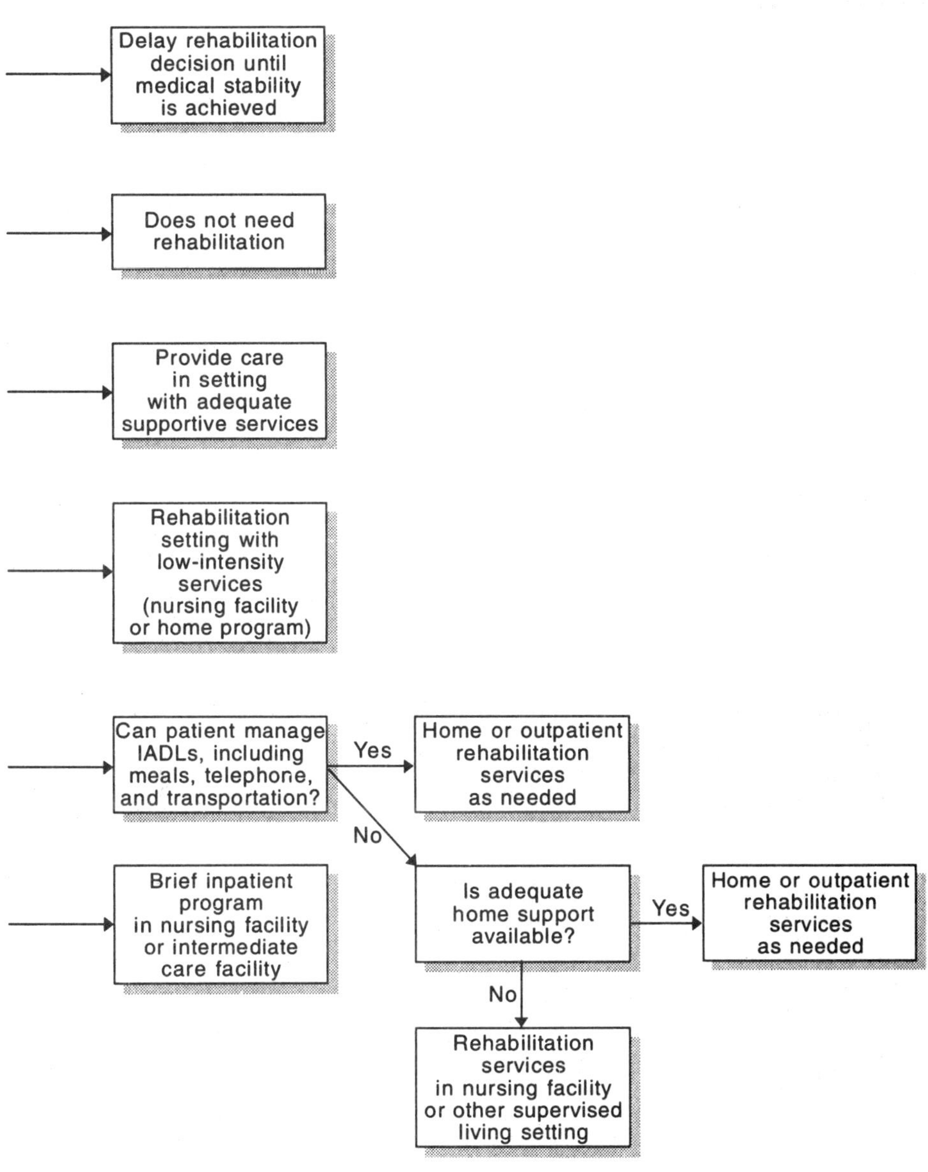
Delay rehabilitation decision until medical stability is achieved
Does not need rehabilitation
Provide care in setting with adequate supportive services
Rehabilitation setting with low-intensity services (nursing facility or home program)
Can patient manage IADLs, including meals, telephone, and transportation?
Yes
Home or outpatient rehabilitation services as needed
No
Brief inpatient program in nursing facility or intermediate care facility
Is adequate home support available?
Yes
Home or outpatient rehabilitation services as needed
No
Rehabilitation services in nursing facility or other supervised living setting

Recommendation: Patients who are medically unstable are generally not suitable for any type of rehabilitation program. Patients who are moderately stable but have complex medical problems that require continuous monitoring are usually better treated in inpatient rehabilitation facilities that not only have 24-hour coverage by physicians and nurses skilled in rehabilitation, but also immediately available consultation services from other medical specialties. (Research evidence=NA; expert opinion=strong consensus.)

Few rehabilitation settings have the capability to manage patients who are acutely ill or medically unstable. Patients who develop acute problems during rehabilitation, including worsening of the stroke or a new stroke, will often require transfer to an acute facility that can adequately treat the problem. An exception would be a rehabilitation program that is so closely linked to an acute care facility that adequate diagnosis and treatment can be provided without transfer. This type of linkage is more likely if the rehabilitation program is located in or adjacent to an acute care hospital.

Inpatient rehabilitation facilities that are certified by CARF and JCAHO are required to have 24-hour coverage by skilled rehabilitation physicians and nurses. Coverage in nursing facilities, even those with "intense" programs, is variable and usually less comprehensive. Intense home programs, while they have skilled rehabilitation physicians and nurses on staff, serve the patient on an intermittent or "on-call" basis. Hence, the patient who requires close observation to detect incipient problems, or frequent adjustment of medications, is better suited for a rehabilitation hospital or unit.

Recommendation: Patients who meet threshold criteria and need moderate to total assistance in mobility or performing basic activities of daily living are candidates for an intense rehabilitation program, if they are able to tolerate 3 or more hours of physical activity each day, or less intense programs if they are not. (Research evidence=C; expert opinion=consensus.)

Evidence suggests, but does not establish, that more intense rehabilitation leads to more rapid improvement and better long-term outcomes than more slowly paced programs (see Table 10). Two controlled studies that involved outpatient therapy found positive relationships between the intensity of therapy and functional outcomes in patients with mild or moderate levels of impairment (Smith, Goldenberg, Ashburn, et al., 1981; Sunderland, Tinson, Bradley, et al., 1992 and 1994). Similarly, two studies of inpatient rehabilitation found that more intense therapy on specialized units led to better functional outcomes than care on general medical units (Sivenius, Pyorala, Heinonen, et al., 1985; Stevens, Ambler, and Warren, 1984). Only Smith, Goldenberg, Ashburn, et al. (1981), however, clearly separated the intensity of therapy from other differences in treatments that may have influenced outcomes. It is difficult to extrapolate the results of these studies to other patient populations or other rehabilitation settings. Nonetheless, there is an inference that "more is better," at least for patients with moderate levels of disability.

As previously discussed, intense rehabilitation can be provided in an inpatient rehabilitation unit or hospital, selected nursing facilities, or selected home programs. The choice depends on the desired degree of intensity and the patient's medical needs. Even nursing facilities and home care providers with "intense" programs usually do not provide the same level of services as a rehabilitation hospital. The availability and commitment of a caregiver to support the patient and participate in rehabilitation are critical to providing intense home-based rehabilitation.

The choice of rehabilitation program for patients needing moderate to total physical assistance will depend on their ability to tolerate the physical activity required by rehabilitation. Patients who can tolerate 3 or more hours of activity a day, or would be expected to do so within a few days in the program, are candidates for an intense rehabilitation program; while those who tolerate only lower levels of activity are usually better served by more slowly paced programs in a nursing facility, an outpatient facility, or the home.

An important consideration is that the energy costs of a physical activity are directly related to the severity of motor disabilities. Hence, a patient with reduced physical activity endurance but less severe motor disability may be able to tolerate intense therapy, while a patient with similar endurance but a more severe disability may not. Some patients who initially have limited physical endurance will improve sufficiently to permit more intense therapy at a later time.

Recommendation: Patients who meet threshold criteria and require only supervision or minimal assistance in mobility or ADL are usually candidates for home or outpatient rehabilitation if the home environment and support are adequate, or for a nursing facility if they are not. (Research evidence=NA; expert opinion=consensus.)

This recommendation applies to patients who are only mildly disabled but are not able to live independently. Safety as well as performance of the essential ADL are concerns. Some patients who need only minimal assistance may be appropriate for inpatient hospital or nursing facility programs if they have complex, multiple functional deficits from physical and/or cognitive impairments, even if home support is adequate. A relatively brief period of rehabilitation in an inpatient program that is targeted at specific disabilities may be sufficient to permit people to live independently.

Recommendation: Patients who have a mild functional deficit but are able to live independently and manage both basic and more complex activities of daily living may benefit from selected rehabilitation

services, but do not require an interdisciplinary rehabilitation program. (Research evidence=NA; expert opinion=consensus.)

People who do not require assistance in ambulation or in performing basic personal care activities may still have difficulty performing more complex activities such as housekeeping, meal preparation, use of public transportation, leisure activities, or returning to work. Furthermore, some people may have communication problems but no motor deficits. Rehabilitation services targeted at problem areas may help to increase independence and improve quality of life for those patients, but an interdisciplinary program is rarely needed. Services can be provided on an outpatient basis or at home if a person has adequate support. If, however, a person does not have adequate support, services can be provided in a nursing facility or other supervised living setting.

6 Managing Rehabilitation

Introduction

This chapter describes the principles and processes of rehabilitation for patients who are admitted to an interdisciplinary program in any type of setting: inpatient hospital rehabilitation facilities, nursing facilities, outpatient or day hospital facilities, and home-based programs. The complexity, intensity, and duration of services vary among settings, but the principles and processes are similar. The focus is on the patient who enters a rehabilitation program following an acute hospitalization for stroke. It is recognized that many patients will require a continuum of care involving movement from one level to another as recovery proceeds. These transitions often reflect a cost-effective use of rehabilitation resources. The present discussion establishes a framework for the initial rehabilitation program, but many of the same considerations apply to later stages and to people with mild deficits who receive rehabilitation services from a single provider.

Preventing complications of stroke is just as important during rehabilitation as it is during the acute hospitalization. The reader is referred to Chapter 4 for a discussion of preventing complications.

Principles of Rehabilitation

Rehabilitation seeks to help the person with disabilities achieve the highest possible degree of physical and psychological performance. To these ends, rehabilitation is both a philosophy and a set of tasks; a rehabilitation program is comparable to school in which the patient is provided an opportunity for instruction, support, protected practice, education, reassurance, direct assistance, and feedback. Rehabilitation has been aptly described as "the planned withdrawal of support," in which services are provided when needed and removed when no longer needed (Roth, 1988). Intrinsic features are involvement of the patient and family in setting goals and planning and implementing treatments, and systematic withdrawal of assistance and return of control to the patient (Charness, 1986; Hyams, 1969). Rehabilitation is done *with* the patient rather than *to* the patient.

Brandstater and Basmajian (1987) and Roth (1988) identify the following common features of comprehensive stroke rehabilitation programs:

- Commitment to continuity of care from the acute phase of the stroke through long-term followup.
- Use of an interdisciplinary team of professionals experienced in and dedicated to the care of the patient with stroke.

- Careful attention to the prevention, recognition, and treatment of comorbid illnesses and intercurrent medical complications.
- Early initiation of goal-directed treatment that takes maximal advantage of the patient's abilities and minimizes disabilities.
- Emphasis on skills development and functional enhancement through training, demonstration, supervision, practice, and appropriate feedback.
- Systematic assessment of the patient's progress during rehabilitation, with adjustment of treatment to maximize benefits.
- Emphasis on patient and family/caregiver education.
- Attention to psychological and social issues affecting both the patient and family/caregiver.
- Early and comprehensive discharge planning aimed at a smooth transition to the community, and at continuity of care to promote social reintegration and resumption of roles in the home, family, recreational, and vocational domains.

Rehabilitation treatments aim to reduce impairments (remediation) or to help patients relearn old skills or develop new ones despite persisting neurological deficits (compensation). Patient and family education, emotional support, psychological counseling, recreational therapy, vocational counseling, and orthotics may also make important contributions. Throughout rehabilitation, attention needs to be directed to the carryover of skills that are learned to different settings. For example, skills learned in an ideal rehabilitation environment often have to be adapted to circumstances existing in a permanent place of residence.

Transition From the Acute Care Hospital

The challenges faced by the patient and family depend on whether the patient returns home to receive rehabilitation there or in an outpatient facility or is transferred to an inpatient rehabilitation hospital or nursing facility for rehabilitation. In either case, adjustment may be difficult.

A return to a familiar environment has distinct advantages, but it also involves a marked reduction of professional support and requires the patient and family to assume responsibility for daily functions and continued recovery. Most outpatient or home rehabilitation programs are limited to a few hours 3 or 4 days a week and are of fairly low intensity. Exceptions are the intense day hospital or home rehabilitation programs that are available in some communities. Chapter 7 discusses the issues that arise during the transition to community living.

Transfer to an inpatient or nursing facility rehabilitation program can also be difficult. These settings offer the advantage of more professional support, as well as support from other patients, which often helps to reduce anxiety and strengthen motivation. However, the people, environment, and procedures encountered in rehabilitation settings are very different from those of the acute hospital and may be confusing at first. Prompt and thorough orientation of patients and families, sensitivity to their concerns, and ample time devoted to addressing questions facilitate adjustment. Rehabilitation is a learning experience that works best when the patient is at ease, the environment is conductive to learning, and the training is focused.

Recommendation: A complete record of medical information from the acute care hospital should be available at the time of admission to any type of rehabilitation program. Significant discrepancies between these records and current clinical findings should be identified and addressed immediately. (Research evidence=NA; expert opinion=strong consensus.)

Transfer to any type of rehabilitation setting requires the prompt transfer of complete medical information including the discharge summary from the acute hospital, results of the rehabilitation screening examination, and current medications. This information should accompany the patient or be sent in advance. Rehabilitation staff should review these records on the day of admission to detect any new problems, significant discrepancies in clinical findings, or urgent questions about treatment regimens. Patients with a stroke usually have medical problems in addition to stroke, and even those who were considered medically stable at the time of transfer are at risk of untoward changes in their condition.

Managing the Rehabilitation Process

A well-conceived rehabilitation management plan is the foundation of a rehabilitation program. This should reflect the priorities expressed by the patient and family, should be based on the results of a baseline clinical assessment of medical conditions and neurological deficits, and should be consistent with the capabilities of the particular rehabilitation setting. The rehabilitation plan includes a clear description of the patient's impairments, disabilities, and strengths; explicit statements of short-term and long-term functional goals; and specification of treatment strategies to achieve the goals. Priorities need to be clearly established among goals, especially in patients with multiple complex deficits.

A schematic diagram of the steps in developing the rehabilitation management plan is shown in Figure 6. Monitoring progress and reevaluating treatment goals and strategies are essential features.

Baseline Assessment on Admission to a Rehabilitation Program

Timing and Content

Recommendation: A complete baseline assessment by the rehabilitation team should be completed for most patients within 3 working days

Figure 6. Development of a rehabilitation management plan

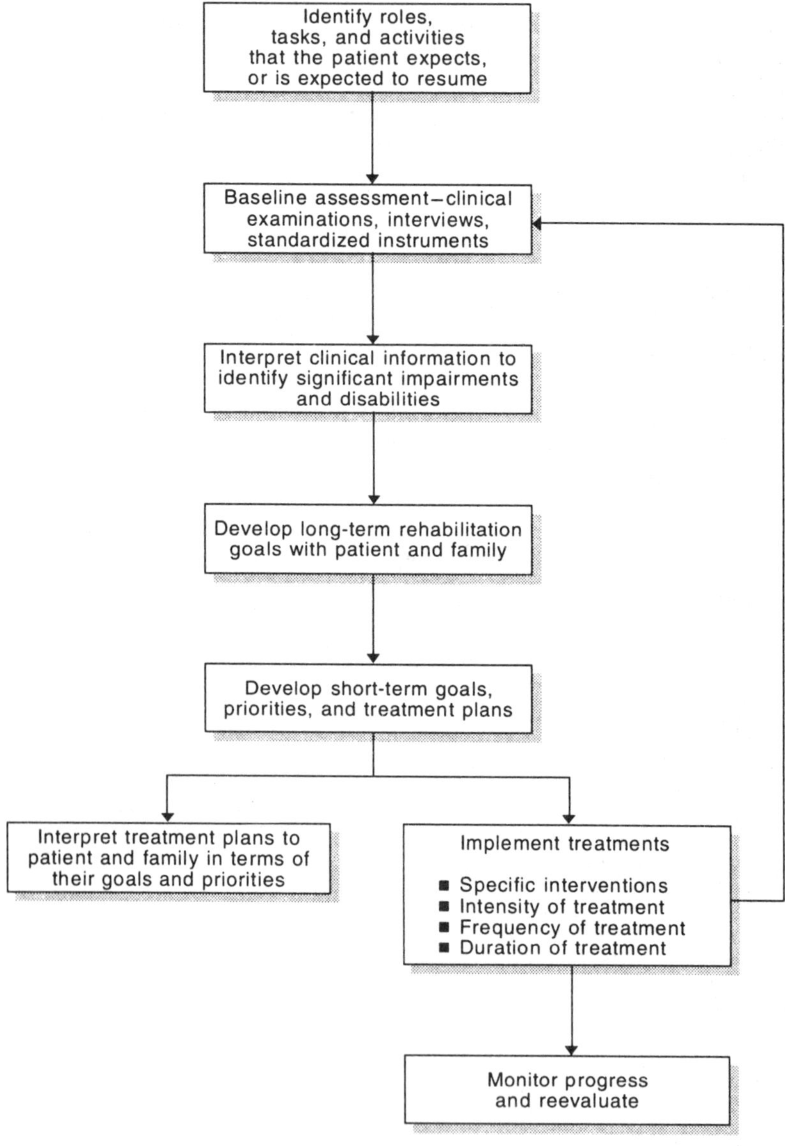

after admission to an intense rehabilitation program in an inpatient rehabilitation facility or nursing facility, within 1 week of admission to a low-intensity nursing facility program, or within three visits for an outpatient or home rehabilitation program. Initial evaluation by a physician and a nurse, including medical and neurological examinations and development of a medical care plan, should be completed within 24 hours of admission or, in the case of outpatient and home programs, on the first visit. All information should be fully documented in the patient's record. (Research evidence=NA; expert opinion=consensus.)

The baseline assessment reaffirms the referral decision, provides the information needed to develop rehabilitation goals and a management plan, and serves as the starting point for monitoring progress. The recommended content is summarized in Table 12.

Evaluation by a physician and a nurse on the day of admission to an inpatient rehabilitation program is essential to determine the patient's current clinical status, identify current medications, assess ability to perform basic ADL (such as feeding, toileting, and transfers), observe behavioral patterns, and identify safety risks. Home and outpatient rehabilitation programs should perform this initial evaluation during the first visit. Any discrepancies with the acute hospital's records should be noted and resolved as soon as possible. A thorough medical history, medical and neurological examinations, and evaluation of functional health patterns provide the foundation. Particular attention should be paid to detecting signs of incipient complications such as DVT, recurrent stroke, or skin breakdown.

The use of standardized instruments facilitates reliable documentation of functional disabilities. This helps to increase the consistency of treatment decisions, facilitates communication among therapists, and provides a reliable basis for monitoring progress. A stroke deficit scale and a mental status screening test need not be repeated if they were administered during a recent rehabilitation screening examination, unless findings of the neurological examination suggest changes in levels of impairment. A broad-based disability scale should be used with all patients. The choice of specific impairment measures will depend on the deficits of the individual patient.

The 3-day, 1-week, or three-visit limit for completing the baseline assessment reflects both cost and quality of care considerations. These limits, though somewhat shorter than the norm of current practice, are reasonable for all except the most complex patients. People with multiple deficits in sensorimotor, cognitive, perceptual, language, and behavioral areas may require longer periods of evaluation.

Table 12. Baseline assessment on admission to a rehabilitation program

Historical information
■ Discharge summary from acute hospitalization. ■ Complete profile from screening examination.
General clinical assessment: neurological and medical examinations and selected laboratory tests
■ Type(s) and severity of neurological deficits and disabilities. ■ Type(s) and severity of comorbid diseases. ■ Complications of stroke. ■ Functional health patterns: nutrition and hydration, ability to swallow, bowel and bladder function, skin integrity, activity tolerance, sleep patterns. ■ Functional status prior to stroke.
Social and environmental factors[a]
■ Presence of spouse or significant other. ■ Previous living situation. ■ Ethnicity and native language. ■ Adjustments of patient and family to stroke. ■ Patient and family preferences for and expectations of rehabilitation. ■ Extent of support by family or involved others (relationships, number, health, availability). ■ Characteristics of potential postdischarge environments.
Standardized instruments (numbers in parentheses refer to attachment tables in this guideline)
■ Stroke deficit scale (2) and mental status screening (5) if not done as part of the screening examination. ■ Impairment measures (individualized to patient's deficits): - Motor function (6). - Mobility (8). - Balance (7). - Language and speech (9). ■ Measure of disability (ADL) (4). ■ Family assessment (12).

[a]For information on social and environmental factors, see Table 5 in Chapter 3.

Note: ADL = activities of daily living.

Evaluating Disabilities

Recommendation: A well-standardized measure of disabilities in basic ADL should be administered to all patients by a rehabilitation professional who is skilled in its use. (Research evidence=NA; expert opinion=strong consensus.)

The primary goal of rehabilitation is to improve functional capability of patients. The two instruments described in Attachment 4 are the most widely used and best validated of those available.

Evaluating Motor Function

Recommendation: Baseline assessment of motor function should include thorough evaluation of motor control and muscle strength, mobility, balance, and coordination (using standardized instruments). Assessment should be performed by professionals who are experienced in rehabilitation and the evaluation of neurological impairments and the completion of these instruments. (Research evidence=NA; expert opinion=strong consensus.)

Complete, accurate, and reliable documentation of motor impairments is essential to successful rehabilitation. The recommendation stresses the major ingredients. Impairments should be documented using standardized instruments such as those described in Attachments 6, 7, and 8.

Evaluating Cognitive Function

Recommendation: A clinical psychological examination should be performed in patients who show evidence of cognitive or emotional problems on clinical examination or a mental status screening test. Complete neuropsychological testing is required when more precise understanding of deficits will facilitate treatment. (Research evidence=NA; expert opinion=consensus.)

The incidence of cognitive deficits and emotional disorders in stroke patients is high (Hibbard and Gordon, 1992; Schubert, Taylor, Lee, et al., 1992a). Cognitive deficits are often associated with longer lengths of stay in rehabilitation programs and with poorer functional outcomes (Galski, Bruno, Zorowitz, et al., 1993; Hier and Edelstein, 1991; Jongbloed, 1986).

A clinical psychological evaluation should sample key cognitive, emotional, behavioral, and motivational domains. Cognitive elements include attention, orientation, memory, language, reasoning, judgment, spatial skills, motor coordination, and social skills. By far, the most common emotional disturbance after a stroke is depression (see Chapter 6). Motivation refers to awareness of deficits and their consequences, attitudes toward rehabilitation, and the level of energy that a patient is able and willing to commit.

A typical examination will require 1 to 2 hours by a mental health professional. Goals are to obtain a profile of the patient's strengths and weaknesses and to identify areas that require attention during rehabilitation or further neuropsychological testing. A neuropsychological examination may be helpful in determining the location of specific brain damage and its implications for treatment. This guideline leaves the selection of instruments or batteries to the discretion of the neuropsychologist.

Evaluating Communicative Function

Recommendation: Patients with problems in functional communication on routine testing should be evaluated using a motor-speech examination, a functional assessment of language and communication abilities, and selected standardized tests. Assessment should be performed by a professional who is experienced in the evaluation of speech and language disorders and in the administration of these instruments. (Research evidence=NA; expert opinion=consensus.)

Speech and language disorders may significantly interfere with the patient's ability to participate in rehabilitation or to return to an independent and fulfilling life. A thorough and accurate assessment of underlying deficits is essential to effective treatment planning. Suggested standardized instruments are listed in Attachment 9.

Evaluating Family/Caregiver Support and the Living Environment

Recommendation: Assessment of family and potential caregiver support and of the living environment is an important part of baseline assessment. A well-standardized instrument should be used when applicable. (Research evidence=NA; expert opinion=strong consensus.)

The patient's support system and contextual factors concerning the patient, family or involved others, and potential living environments (see Table 6 and Attachment 12) should be evaluated at the time of admission to rehabilitation and again before discharge. Rehabilitation requires full knowledge of the personal and physical environments in which the patient will be functioning. Use of an instrument, such as the Family Assessment Device, is recommended with patients who have families (spouse or other). This instrument has been used extensively with stroke patients and has a well-demonstrated ability to identify family characteristics relating to problem solving, roles, communication, affect, behavior control, and general functioning.

Setting Rehabilitation Goals

Recommendation: Both short-term and longer term goals need to be realistic in terms of current levels of disability and the potential for recovery. Goals should be mutually agreed to by the patient, family, and rehabilitation team and should be documented in the medical record in explicit, measurable terms. (Research evidence=NA; expert opinion=strong consensus.)

Overly ambitious goals for rehabilitation will set the patient (and family) up for failure and may lead to unwarranted use of rehabilitation facilities. However, goals that are too modest may not make full use of the patient's potential.

Four considerations are especially important. First, recovery after stroke is highly variable and only partly predictable. Even carefully conceived goals may be inaccurate. For this reason, goals that are set at the time of admission to a rehabilitation program need to be reevaluated at regular intervals and modified to reflect the rate of a patient's progress.

Second, the time since stroke onset is important. Recovery due to neurological healing is most rapid during the first 1 to 3 months after a stroke and then plateaus. Significant functional improvement is less common after 6 months, although it can occur (Kelly-Hayes, Wolf, Kase, et al., 1989; Skilbeck, Wade, Hewer, et al., 1983). Expectations for further improvement might therefore be more optimistic in a patient with a recent stroke and a favorable initial recovery trajectory—than in a patient whose stroke occurred 2 or 3 months before—or one who has improved little during the post-stroke period.

Third, rehabilitation goals need to take into account patient characteristics that have been associated with poor functional prognoses (see Chapter 2). For example, persistent urinary incontinence often portends a poor outcome. The absence of any volitional movement in a limb 2 to 4 weeks after a stroke suggests that significant neurological recovery is unlikely, and that rehabilitation goals might better be focused on training in compensatory techniques, or the use of adaptive equipment.

Finally, rehabilitation goals need to address the full range of factors that influence functional performance, including psychological and social adjustment and physical conditioning.

Developing the Rehabilitation Management Plan

Recommendation: The rehabilitation management plan should indicate the specific treatments planned and their sequence, intensity, frequency, and expected duration. Measures to prevent complications of stroke and recurrent strokes should be continued. (Research evidence=NA except for some preventive measures; expert opinion=strong consensus.)

As a general principle, medical problems or complications of stroke that increase patient risk or interfere with rehabilitation should be addressed first. Examples include congestive heart failure, urinary tract infections, and musculoskeletal pain. High priority is also given to the prevention of thromboembolism and recurrent stroke (as discussed in Chapter 4), and the maintenance of functional health patterns such as nutrition and bowel and bladder control.

Rehabilitation therapies then target impairments in mobility and motor control and disabilities in ADL performance. Treatments for depression or other emotional problems, perceptual deficits, and speech and language problems are added in patients who need them.

Decisions on the intensity and frequency of interventions depend heavily on the patient's physical endurance, level of motivation, and attention span. The patient's ability to tolerate physical activity will often be limited by preexisting health problems, age-related physiologic changes, or deconditioning effects of immobility (Mol and Baker, 1991). As discussed in Chapter 3, there is currently no standard approach to evaluating physical activity endurance. Patients with severe limitations in exercise tolerance may be best served by a slowly paced program or even by delaying rehabilitation until after a further period of recuperation.

The patient's motivation to participate in rehabilitation is also an important consideration. Assessment of motivation is complex and imprecise. Apparent motivational problems may actually reflect communication deficits or lack of clarity in instructions by staff. Poor motivation may be due to modifiable causes such as depression, incongruence between the patient's goals and those of the rehabilitation program, or a failure of the rehabilitation team to make clear the connection between interventions and goals that are valued by the patient. Motivation may also be affected by neurological deficits that lead to hypoarousal, apathy, or a lack of awareness of disabilities. Mood or memory disorders are especially likely to be denied by patients (Anderson and Tranel, 1989; Hibbard, Gordon, Stein, et al., 1992).

The family may play a pivotal role in helping to identify depressive symptoms or areas of misunderstanding or dissatisfaction with the rehabilitation program and may also help the patient cope with the effects of the stroke and develop the motivation to make a maximal effort to recover (Phipps, 1990). If, despite all efforts, the patient is not able to participate actively, rehabilitation may have to be deferred.

The Interdisciplinary Team Approach

The varied and complex manifestations of stroke often require the services of specialists from several disciplines. The team approach facilitates coordination of care; simultaneous treatment of motor, cognitive, and speech and language deficits; and tailoring of treatment schedules to the patient's priorities and responses to treatment.

Composition of the team varies with the patient's needs and the available resources. In comprehensive inpatient programs, participants include a physician expert in rehabilitation, a rehabilitation nurse, a physical therapist, an occupational therapist, a clinical psychologist, a social worker, and often a therapeutic recreation specialist. A speech-language pathologist will often become involved if the patient has speech, language, or swallowing problems. Other participants may include a psychiatrist, other medical or surgical specialists, and a physician assistant, respiratory therapist, registered dietitian, vocational counselor, chaplain, orthotist, or rehabilitation engineer.

Effective teamwork is not easy. Conflicts arise when communication breaks down or when differences of opinions or interpretations of the patient's behavior are not resolved (Rothberg, 1981). Strong leadership, clarity of roles and responsibilities, and a willingness to devote time and effort to communication are essential. The team leader, who may be from any discipline, is the central figure and assumes primary responsibility for coordinating services and facilitating communication among team members, the patient, and the family. Team conferences, frequent contacts among team members, and complete and intelligible entries in the patient's medical record are important.

The conceptual appeal of the team approach for coordinating stroke care has led to its widespread adoption. However, concrete evidence supporting its effectiveness and cost effectiveness is limited. A literature review concluded that team care resulted in better control or less deterioration in patients with chronic illnesses—but also in more utilization of health services and higher costs (Halstead, 1976). Controlled studies of team care in stroke rehabilitation are limited to the previously discussed (see Chapter 4) stroke unit studies, in which the "team" is one aspect of a multidimensional intervention. Ultimately, the greater expense of the team approach needs to be justified by documentation of greater patient benefits.

Implementation Principles

The Learning Process

Recommendation: Rehabilitation should follow well-supported principles of effective learning. (Research evidence=C; expert opinion=strong consensus.)

Rehabilitation is predominantly a learning process. Adherence to basic principles of learning requires that:

- Careful assessment is done to determine tasks that a patient can perform.
- The skills or knowledge being taught are meaningful to the patient.
- Training is graded by level of difficulty, and less complex or demanding tasks are addressed first, so that the patients can experience success.
- Instructions are phrased as concretely as possible and are short, direct, and simple.
- Instructions are understood.
- Tasks to be mastered or information to be learned are tailored to the person's abilities in order to avoid "overload."
- Steps are taken to slow patient responses if impulsivity causes a person to perform a task too rapidly or unsafely.
- Feedback on performance is provided by the therapist or by use of videotapes to reinforce desired responses.
- Steps are taken to stimulate responses (e.g., by timing the patient in the performance of a task or by talking about favorite activities) in order to overcome periods of hypoarousal or lethargy.

- Repetition and practice are used between training sessions when the patient is on the unit or at home.

Application of these principles should take account of the patient's current abilities and should be adjusted in response to improvements over the course of rehabilitation.

Family Involvement

Recommendation: Families or involved others should be active participants in the rehabilitation process. (Research evidence=NA; expert opinion=strong consensus.)

Family involvement in the rehabilitation process includes encouraging the free expression of questions, concerns, and ideas; participation in the development of rehabilitation goals and the management plan; the opportunity to validate expectations of rehabilitation against the realities of patient progress; and "hands-on" participation in therapy sessions. The family can, and should, serve as an active advocate for the patient throughout the rehabilitation process. Easy access to information will help allay the family's anxieties and build a partnership toward understanding and confronting the patient's disabilities. Active participation of family members in therapy sessions provides encouragement to the patient at the same time as it helps to develop the skills needed to assist the patient at home.

Patient and Family Education

Recommendation: Patients, families, and involved others should be given information and provided with ample opportunity to learn about the causes and consequences of stroke and the goals, process, and prognosis of rehabilitation. Family members and other potential caregivers should receive thorough training in techniques and problem-solving approaches required to provide effective support. (Research evidence=B; expert opinion=strong consensus.)

Patient and family education is an integral part of rehabilitation. It greatly contributes to achieving improved outcomes (Evans, Matlock, Bishop, et al., 1988). Education begun during the acute hospitalization is reinforced early and often during rehabilitation through discussions among the patient, family, and therapists; didactic sessions; family participation in therapy sessions; and the use of books, brochures, and videotapes. Potential topics are listed in Table 13.

Education should be adapted to the educational and cultural background of the patient and family, the mental status of the patient, and emotional factors that may interfere with learning. Experiential learning is often more effective than didactic learning, and repetition is important.

Table 13. Issues for patient and family/caregiver education

What is stroke? ■ Etiology of stroke. ■ Effects of stroke on the patient. ■ Effects of stroke on the family.
Routine care in the hospital, rehabilitation setting, or home ■ Maintenance of nutrition and hydration. ■ Bowel and bladder care. ■ Sleep and rest. ■ Reliable medication taking. ■ Behavioral issues and how to deal with them. ■ Positioning and moving in bed. ■ Prevention of blood clots. ■ Prevention of skin breakdown. ■ Safety measures to prevent falls. ■ Exercise during and after rehabilitation. ■ Techniques for performing specific tasks, such as transfers, personal hygiene, etc. ■ Training in specific skills for which patient needs assistance. ■ Optimizing social functioning.
Complications of stroke (tailored to patient's specific circumstances) ■ Swallowing problems. ■ Care/use of indwelling bladder catheter or feeding tube. ■ Respiratory complications. ■ Care of tracheostomy/use of respiratory equipment. ■ Speech or language deficits; facilitating communication. ■ Depression and other psychological disturbances.
Prevention of recurrent stroke ■ Monitoring blood pressure. ■ Medical or surgical interventions to prevent recurrent stroke. ■ Lifestyle modification.
After hospital care ■ Caregiver concerns. ■ Family functioning. ■ Support groups, respite care. ■ Sexual functioning. ■ Recreational and vocational pursuits. ■ Automobile driving. ■ Vocational counseling.

Counseling and Psychotherapy. For the purposes of this guideline, *counseling* is defined as supportive and educational interventions to assist the patient or family in identifying key issues and problem solving around them. *Psychotherapy* is defined as interventions to change basic mental functions in a person or organizational or transactional patterns in families. Counseling can be provided by a variety of rehabilitation professionals, but psychotherapy is limited to psychiatrists, psychologists, social workers, and psychiatric clinical nurse specialists. Since a recommendation for psychological or social help may be interpreted by patients or their families as an indication that they are somehow deficient, careful assessment and a thorough understanding of the underlying issues should always precede such recommendations. A decision to recommend counseling or psychotherapy should be made only after discussion with the rehabilitation team. Patients and families are able to resolve many problems on their own, without formal counseling, after the problems have been identified and treatment options have been discussed.

Monitoring Progress During Rehabilitation

Recommendation: The patient's progress during rehabilitation should be documented at least weekly during an intense rehabilitation program in an inpatient rehabilitation facility or nursing facility, and at least every other week during less intense nursing facility, outpatient, or home programs. A subset of the standardized measures administered at baseline assessment should be chosen, targeting those impairments and disabilities that have been the focus of treatments during the preceding period. (Research evidence=NA; expert opinion=strong consensus.)

Regular evaluation of progress is needed to obtain the information required to adjust treatment regimens and also to justify continued rehabilitation. Under most circumstances, it is reasonable to expect that measurable (and meaningful) improvement will occur over 1 week during an intense program or over 1 month during a less intense program. An exception would be if rehabilitation were interrupted by an acute illness or for other reasons.

Assessment should include both a clinical examination and a subset of the standardized instruments used during the baseline assessment (see Table 12). Emphasis should be on areas of impairment or function that have been particular targets of interventions during the preceding period. The use of well-standardized, reliable measures is essential to achieving valid comparisons from examination to examination and also comparisons among patients with similar problems. Clinical examinations document changes in medical conditions and areas of progress not addressed by the standardized measures. Regular discussions with family/caregivers can also provide important information on the patient's progress.

Changes in regimens may address specific medical, emotional, or cognitive problems that are impeding physical rehabilitation or may modify the type or intensity of specific treatments or educational interventions.

Preventing Recurrent Stroke and Deep Vein Thrombosis

Prevention of recurrent stroke and prevention of deep vein thrombosis are discussed for the acute care setting in Chapter 4. The same measures continue to apply throughout rehabilitation.

Managing Comorbidities and Acute Illnesses

Associated Medical Conditions

Most patients with strokes have other medical conditions that require treatment during rehabilitation. Severe illnesses may limit the patient's ability to participate in therapeutic exercise and reduce the likelihood of favorable rehabilitation outcomes (Lehmann, DeLateur, Fowler, et al., 1975; Roth, Mueller, and Green, 1988). Common diseases are hypertension, ischemic heart disease, congestive heart failure, chronic pulmonary disease, and diabetes mellitus. Goals of treatment include adjusting antihypertensive medications to control blood pressure while avoiding postural (orthostatic) hypotension, treating angina pectoris and congestive heart failure with medications while adjusting exercise to the patient's abilities, and adjusting diet and medications (insulin, oral agents) in diabetics to accommodate changes in blood sugar that may occur during increased physical activity. A full discussion of the management of these and other comorbidities is beyond the scope of this guideline.

Acute Illnesses

Recommendation: A patient who develops an acute medical illness during rehabilitation should be evaluated promptly and, if necessary, transferred to an acute care facility. (Research evidence=NA; expert opinion=strong consensus.)

Few rehabilitation programs have adequate diagnostic or treatment capabilities to care for acute medical illnesses such as acute myocardial infarction, pulmonary embolus, or gastrointestinal bleeding. These patients will require transfer to an acute care facility. Close cross-coverage arrangements with an acute care facility will, in some cases, reduce the need for transfer. The ability of rehabilitation facilities to care for other acute (but less life-threatening) illnesses such as urinary tract infection, pneumonia, or thrombophlebitis, varies widely. Decisions on the need for transfer should be individualized to the capabilities of the program. In general, rehabilitation programs should have a low threshold for obtaining consultations or initiating transfer when acute problems arise.

Managing Functional Health Patterns

Managing Dysphagia

The assessment of swallowing disorders (dysphagia) is discussed in Chapter 3, and management is discussed in Chapter 4. Swallowing problems frequently resolve spontaneously; however, the condition should be reassessed at the time of admission to rehabilitation and treatments continued or modified, if necessary.

Maintaining Nutrition and Hydration

Recommendation: The adequacy of the oral intake of food and fluids should be monitored regularly. (Research evidence=NA; expert opinion=strong consensus.)

A significant number of patients have evidence of dehydration or inadequate nutrition at the time of admission with a stroke, and one report indicates that as many as 22 percent of patients evidence deficiencies by the time of discharge (Axelsson, Asplund, Norberg, et al., 1988). Possible causes of inadequate oral intake are dysphagia, an inability to chew or feed oneself, lack of interest in food, cognitive deficits such as inability to recognize hunger or thirst, and inability to make hunger or thirst known because of problems with communication. Possible effects are generalized weakness, increased risk of skin breakdown and pressure ulcers, electrolyte imbalance, and reduced ability to participate in rehabilitation.

To reduce the risk of malnutrition or dehydration, food and fluid intake should be monitored daily in all patients, and body weight should be determined regularly. Opportunities to improve intake include catering to a patient's food preferences, arranging for company during meals, providing assistance in feeding or otherwise encouraging intake, and treating specific problems that interfere with intake. If such measures are unsuccessful, feeding by a feeding gastrostomy may be necessary.

Managing Bladder Function

Recommendation: Persistent urinary incontinence after a stroke should be evaluated to determine its etiology, and cause-specific treatment should be implemented. (Research evidence=C; expert opinion=strong consensus.)

Urinary incontinence that persists after a stroke is often associated with severe motor, proprioceptive, and visual deficits and a poor long-term prognosis (Reding, Winter, Hochrein, et al., 1987). Causes include damage to neural centers that govern bladder function, immobility that prevents timely access to toileting facilities, cognitive deficits that prevent recognition of the need to void, and communication problems that interfere with making needs known to others. Fecal impaction may also predispose to incontinence by causing pressure on the bladder. Potential complications include urinary tract infection, skin breakdown, social embarrassment, depression, and the need for institutionalization.

Documentation of the duration and pattern of urinary incontinence should include frequency of urination, timing, amount, whether voiding was preceded by the urge to urinate, discomfort on voiding (dysuria), and fluid intake patterns.

Management is cause-specific. In most cases, efforts should be made to remove an indwelling catheter, if one has been placed, in conjunction with a bladder training program that includes timed voiding and use of a commode or toilet instead of a bedpan. Intermittent catheterization may be indicated if postvoid residual volumes (PVR) greater than 50 cc are associated with symptomatic urinary tract infections. However, many patients tolerate increased PVRs without developing urinary tract infections and do not require intermittent catheterization. Bladder training is especially useful in patients who are alert and cooperative but may also be helpful in the cognitively impaired patient (Engel, Burgio, McCormick, et al., 1990; McCormick, Scheve, and Leahy, 1988; Schnelle, 1990). A clamping regimen prior to removal of an indwelling catheter does not appear to be helpful (Gross, 1990). Attention by staff to voiding needs and adequate access to toileting facilities are both essential.

Patient and family education in the management of bladder function is an important part of discharge planning.

Managing Bowel Function

Recommendation: Bowel management programs should be implemented in patients with persistent constipation or bowel incontinence. (Research evidence=B; expert opinion=consensus.)

Fecal incontinence occurs in a substantial proportion of patients after a stroke but clears within 2 weeks in the majority (Brocklehurst, Andrews, Richards, et al., 1985). Continued fecal incontinence signals a poor prognosis. Diarrhea, when it occurs, may be due to medications, initiation of tube feedings, or infection. It can also be due to leakage around a fecal impaction. Treatment should be cause-specific.

Constipation and fecal impaction are more common after stroke than incontinence. Immobility and inactivity, inadequate fluid or food intake, depression or anxiety, a neurogenic bowel or the inability to perceive bowel signals, lack of transfer ability, and cognitive deficits may each contribute. Goals of management are to ensure adequate intake of fluid, bulk, and fiber and to help the patient establish a regular toileting schedule. Bowel training is more effective if the schedule is consistent with the patient's previous bowel habits (Venn, Taft, Carpentier, et al., 1992). Stool softeners and judicious use of laxatives may be helpful.

Managing Sleep Disturbances

Recommendation: Sleep disturbances should be assessed and indicated changes for sleep habits, environment, or medications should be implemented as necessary. (Research evidence=NA; expert opinion=strong consensus.)

Sleep patterns may be altered by the effects of the stroke or by routines of a hospital or nursing facility. Inverted sleep-wake rhythms with lethargy during daytime hours and agitation at night, sleep apnea (Culebras, 1992), and reduced sleep efficiency with a suppression of REM sleep and increased non-REM sleep (Korner, Flooh, Reinhart, et al., 1986) have been reported to result from hemisphere strokes. Depression or anxiety may interfere with sleep (Chenelly, 1989). Muscle spasms, pain, inability to move in bed, and urinary frequency or incontinence can interrupt sleep. The unfamiliar environment of a hospital, noise, and awakenings for medications or vital signs also create problems for some patients (Beyerman, 1987).

Lack of adequate sleep can interfere with a patient's ability to participate in an intense rehabilitation schedule. Daytime rest periods may be needed because of fatigue due to vigorous activities, but these must be weighed against the ability of the patient to sleep at night.

Assessment of sleep problems includes the patient's sleep history, observation of sleep and waking behaviors, evaluation of medications, and examination of environmental factors. Management should address the cause of the sleep problem and treat the appropriate disability or symptom; change the environment to reduce disturbances during sleep or adjust the type, timing, and dose of the offending medication. Hypnotics should be used only if all else fails. In this regard, a small controlled trial found that flurazepam produced more daytime sedation than triazolam in patients with strokes (Woo, Proulx, and Greenblatt, 1991).

If sleep medications are used, side effects such as daytime sedation, paradoxical agitation, confusion, or memory problems need to be carefully monitored. Moreover, there is suggestive evidence that agents such as benzodiazepines may slow sensorimotor recovery (Goldstein, 1993), and these agents should be used only if all else fails. Interventions to keep the patient active and minimize daytime sleep, relaxation and other behavioral techniques to help induce sleep, and devices to prevent sleep apnea should also be considered.

Managing Sensorimotor Deficits and Impaired Mobility

Introduction

Sensorimotor deficits and restricted physical mobility are common after stroke. These problems may be complex in their own right and are made even more so by coexisting cardiovascular disease, arthritis, or physical deconditioning. A patient's movement problems may involve muscle weakness, abnormal synergistic organization of movements, altered temporal sequencing of muscle contractions, impaired regulation of force control, delayed responses, abnormal muscle tone, loss of range of motion, altered biomechanical alignment, and sensory impairments.

The first challenge facing a therapist is to determine which factors are contributing to movement or functional deficits. Assessment begins by observing a patient's attempts to accomplish functional tasks. Apparent disabilities are then examined using standardized measures of deficits in movement, posture, and physical performance. Thorough knowledge of the cause of impaired motor performance is needed to select appropriate exercises, treatment modalities, and activities.

The three philosophies that guide treatment choices for sensorimotor deficits are remediation or facilitation, compensation, and motor control (Duncan, 1992). The remediational approach is exemplified by traditional physical therapy exercises and neuromuscular facilitation. This approach uses forced sensory stimulation modalities, exercises, and resistive training to enhance motor recovery. Some degree of volitional movement in the involved limb is required.

In the compensatory model, the therapist emphasizes achieving independence in basic activities of daily living by attempting to improve function rather than enhancing motor recovery or minimizing impairments. Some therapists avoid the compensatory approach for fear that reliance on the noninvolved side to accomplish daily tasks will suppress recovery and contribute to learned nonuse of the impaired side (Bobath, 1978 and 1990). Evidence supporting this conclusion is provided by studies showing that forced use of the impaired limb improves motor control in some patients (Taub, Miller, Novack, et al., 1993; Wolf, Lecraw, Barton, et al., 1989). However, the compensatory strategy may be the only way to improve function after motor recovery has plateaued. Moreover, it may be preferred in patients with severe motor deficits who have a poor prognosis for recovery of sensorimotor function.

The third model is relatively new and incorporates theories of motor control and motor learning (Carr and Shepherd, 1989; Gordon, 1987; Winstein, 1987). Major tenets of this approach are that motor control represents a complex interaction of the neurological and musculoskeletal systems and the environment to enhance performance. This theory holds that motor control is task-specific, and hence, if one practices under one condition, the effects do not necessarily carry over to another condition. This concept is appealing, but evidence is lacking to support the superiority of treatments based on this view of motor control.

A myriad of therapeutic intervention strategies have been applied in attempts to improve motor control and physical performance. Table 14 provides examples of treatments for different types of impairment. As exemplified by the controlled studies summarized in Table 15, no one type of physical therapy has been shown to be superior to others. Since neuromuscular facilitation treatments are more labor intensive and more expensive than traditional physical therapy, objective proof of their greater effectiveness would be needed to justify their use.

Rehabilitation programs do not typically employ cardiovascular training techniques, but many patients experience some degree of physical conditioning by engaging in rehabilitation activities. Patients with coexisting cardiovascular disease will require evaluation before rehabilitation and monitoring during treatment to minimize the risk of complications. The benefits of incorporating cardiovascular training programs in stroke rehabilitation need to be evaluated.

Exercise and Functional Training for Remediation of Sensorimotor Deficits

Recommendation: Patients who have functional deficits and at least some voluntary control over movements of the involved arm or leg should be encouraged to use the limb in functional tasks and offered exercise and functional training directed at improving strength and motor control, relearning sensorimotor relationships, and improving functional performance. (Research evidence=C; expert opinion=strong consensus.)

Exercise and functional training are indicated if the motor deficit compromises the patient's ability to walk or perform ADL. Published studies report that many patients improve during rehabilitation; however, they do not convincingly establish whether improvement should be attributed to the type, intensity, frequency, and duration of treatment or to spontaneous recovery. The strongest evidence of benefit is from studies that have enrolled patients with chronic deficits or have included a no-treatment control group. For example, Wade found improvement in gait speed after outpatient rehabilitation (Wade, Collen, Robb, et al., 1992), and Smith found a graded response to increasing intensity of outpatient rehabilitation in patients with mild sensorimotor deficits (Smith, Goldenberg, Ashburn, et al., 1981). (See Table 10 in Chapter 5 for a summary of these studies.) Tangeman documented improved balance and ADL performance after functional training in weight-shift balance in patients who were trained a year or more after their stroke (Tangeman,

Table 14. Examples of therapies for sensorimotor deficits and physical mobility

Impairments	Treatments
Sensory deficits	■ Teach compensatory strategies. ■ Patient accommodates to diminished sensory input during movement and functional activities.
Range of motion	■ Passive and active range of motion. ■ Joint mobilization. ■ Splinting or casting.
Pain	■ Positioning (e.g., slings, wheelchair tray, arm supports). ■ Reduction of edema (elevation, pressure gloves or stockings, continuous passive motion, etc.). ■ Modalities (ice, heat, ultrasound, etc.). ■ Proper range of motion (techniques and sequence of exercises to avoid shoulder impingement syndrome).
Force control–voluntary control	■ Facilitory modalities as patient attempts to contract muscles (e.g., quick stretch, vibration, electrical stimulation). ■ Select optimal biomechanical position or position in point of range of motion for patient to initiate movement (e.g., to facilitate hip flexion, have patient assume side lying and place patient's hip in 90 degrees of flexion; also, therapist quick stretches the hip flexors as the patient attempts to contract the muscle). ■ Isometric, eccentric, concentric exercises. ■ Select eccentric exercises prior to concentric exercises. ■ Assistive, active, and resistive exercises. ■ Functional activities (e.g., bridging exercises, sit to stand, dressing, and other daily tasks, etc.). ■ Train the patient in context-specific environments.
Force control–speed	■ Isokinetic exercise training. ■ Functional tasks requiring quick contractions (postural perturbations, kicking a ball, etc.).
Tone–spasticity	■ Stretching, prolonged stretching, passive manipulation by therapists (e.g., slow rhythmic rotation), weight bearing, ice, contraction of muscles antagonistic to spastic muscles, splinting, and casting.
Tone–prolonged recruitment and lack of reciprocal inhibition	■ Exercise muscle groups antagonistic to muscle that will not turn off with the correct timing. ■ Slow active reciprocal contraction of agonist and antagonist muscles.

Table 14. Examples of therapies for sensorimotor deficits and physical mobility (continued)

Impairments	Treatments
Synergistic organization	■ Select exercises, movement patterns, and activities that require increasingly more complex combinations of muscle contractions and sequencing (e.g., ankle dorsiflexion and eversion with hip and knee extended, prehensile patterns of hand with wrist extension, elbow extension, and shoulder flexion). ■ Vary conditions of performance so that patient will be able to adapt to speed and other environmental stresses. ■ Functional use of available controlled movement. ■ Goal is developing a variety of movement patterns and purposeful activities.
Mobility	■ Practice moving in bed, rolling, coming to sit, sit to stand, transfers, standing, walking (activities may be done by encouraging as much use of involved extremities as possible, or patient may be taught to compensate with noninvolved extremities).
Balance	■ Weight-shift training with and without feedback. ■ Selecting activities that require automatic weight transfer (e.g., reaching). ■ Practice a variety of activities under different conditions that require sitting, standing, and walking balance (reaching, turning, changing directions, carrying objects, going up and down hills, catching, throwing, and reaching in various directions). ■ Patient practices restoring balance as his/her balance is perturbed.
Gait	■ Consultation with orthotist to select appropriate orthosis. ■ Select assistive devices. ■ Practice swing, stance, weight shift components with and without feedback from therapists. ■ Vary conditions of performance (speed, sensory conditions, different surfaces).
Impaired ADL	■ Practice all basic activities of daily living (patient may be taught compensatory strategies with or without adaptive equipment). ■ Practice all instrumental activities of daily living that the patient needs to be able to do (telephoning, using checkbook, shopping, etc.). Compensatory strategies with or without adaptive equipment. ■ Practice home and community activities (independent walking in the home and community, home management tasks, etc.).

Table 15. Evidence on the effectiveness of different types of physical therapy

Author Year Country	Purpose Study design Duration of deficits Number of subjects	Outcome measures Maximum followup	Conclusions/ comments
Sunderland, Tinson, Bradley, et al. (1992 and 1994) United Kingdom	Compare enhanced PT to orthodox PT RCT with stratification on side of hemiplegia and severity of upper extremity impairments Acute deficits N=432	Extended Motricity Index Motor Club Assessment Passive movement and pain Frenchay arm test Nine-hole peg test Sensory loss ADL (Barthel) F/U until 1 year	Improved arm function in enhanced therapy group at 6 months that was not sustained at 12 months.
Jongbloed, Stacey, and Brighton (1989) British Columbia	Compare functional and sensorimotor occupational therapies RCT Acute deficits N=90	ADL (Barthel) Meal preparation Sensorimotor Integration Test F/U until 8 weeks	No significant differences among groups.
Dickstein, Hocherman, Pillar, et al. (1986) Israel	Compare 3 therapeutic approaches RCT Acute deficits N=131	ADL (Barthel) Muscle tone Active ROM Strength Ambulatory status F/U until 6 weeks	No significant differences among groups. No difference in functional recovery or stress on caregivers.
Lord and Hall (1986) United States	Compare neuromuscular retraining (NRT) and traditional functional rehabilitation (TFR) Retrospective F/U study with matching Acute deficits N=39	NA F/U until 8 months	No significant differences except NRT improved more on feeding ($p < 0.05$).
Logigian, Samuels, Falconer, et al. (1983) United States	Compare traditional PT and neurofacilitation RCT Acute deficits N=42	ADL (Barthel) Manual Muscle Test F/U until discharge	No differences between groups.

See notes at end of table.

Table 15. Evidence on the effectiveness of different types of physical therapy (continued)

Author Year Country	Purpose Study design Duration of deficits Number of subjects	Outcome measures Maximum followup	Conclusions/ comments
Stern, McDowell, Miller, et al. (1970) United States	Compare neuromuscular reeducation and traditional PT RCT with patients added to "balance" groups Acute deficits N=62	Strength Mobility Index Kenny Self-Care Index F/U until discharge	No differences between groups.

Note: ADL = activities of daily living. F/U = followup. NA = not applicable. PT = physical therapy. RCT = randomized controlled trial. ROM = range of motion.

Banaitis, and Williams, 1990). Using no-treatment control groups in randomized studies, Mandel found that treatment groups that received biofeedback improved more than the control group (Mandel, Nymark, Balmer, et al., 1990). (For more information, see Table 16.)

Patients with mild sensorimotor deficits following stroke may not require any therapeutic intervention. However, evidence from the geriatric literature suggests that accumulated mild deficits in strength, mobility, and coordination contribute to limited physical performance in the elderly (Duncan, Chandler, Studenski, et al., 1993) and increase the risk of falls (Bergstrom, Aniansson, Bjelle, et al., 1985; Jette and Branch, 1981; Lord, Clark, and Webster, 1991; Lundgren-Linquist, Aniansson, and Rundgren, 1983; Studenski, 1992; Studenski, Duncan, and Chandler, 1991; Whipple, Wolfson, and Amerman, 1987). Increasing strength and balance may improve function and reduce falls in these patients (Fiatarone, Marks, Ryan, et al., 1990; Judge, Lindsey, Underwood, et al., 1993; Tinetti, Baker, McAvay, et al., 1994; Tinetti and Ginter, 1988).

Another important issue is that of sustaining levels of function achieved during rehabilitation. Most studies report only short-term outcomes. Those that examine longer-term outcomes reach mixed conclusions. Some of these studies indicate that functional gains are maintained (Indredavik, Bakke, Solberg, et al., 1991; Smith, Goldenberg, Ashburn, et al., 1981; Strand, Asplund, Eriksson, et al., 1985), and others do not (Garraway, Akhtar, Hockey, et al., 1980; Garraway, Akhtar, Prescott, et al., 1980; Garraway, Walton, Akhtar, et al., 1981; Sivenius, Pyorala, Heinonen, et al., 1985; Stevens, Ambler, and Warren, 1984; Sunderland, Tinson, Bradley, et al., 1992 and 1994; Wade, Collen, Robb, et al., 1992). Failures to maintain functional gains appear to underscore the need for continued practice after the patient returns home. The importance of encouragement by family and involved others and the need for the patient to accept progressively more responsibility for independent function can hardly be overemphasized. Continued rehabilitation or "tuneups" may be indicated in some cases, but need to be justified by evidence of progress during treatment and deterioration in its absence.

Evidence on Specific Interventions for Sensorimotor Deficits

Neither research evidence nor expert consensus adequately supports recommendations concerning the superiority of one type of exercise regimen over another, the use of biofeedback or functional electrical stimulation in enhancing responses to functional therapy, the functional benefits of balance retraining, or the use of sensory retraining. The results of controlled studies are summarized in the indicated tables. Conclusions are:

- **Biofeedback.** Results of biofeedback studies (see Table 16) are inconclusive. Two studies have demonstrated sustained functional benefits (Burnside, Tobias, and Bursill, 1982; Mandel, Nymark, Balmer et al., 1990). Other studies have shown transient or no effects. Two meta-analyses have also come to conflicting conclusions. Schleenbaker and Mainous (1993) found that biofeedback is an "effective tool for neuromuscular reeducation" while Glanz, Klawansky, Stason, et al. (1994a) found an insignificant positive effect in pooled studies. Differences in the criteria for selecting studies to be pooled, and differences in the outcome measures used, account for the differing results in these two meta-analyses.
- **Functional electrical stimulation.** Functional electrical stimulation (FES) has been shown to produce short-term increases in muscle strength and motor control in selected patients (see Table 17); however, effects on function have not been adequately studied (Glanz, Klawansky, Stason, et al., 1994b).
- **Balance training.** Computerized biofeedback training designed to improve balance (see Table 18) has been shown to have greater effects on impairment measures (lateral sway, stance symmetry, etc.) than physical therapy alone, but carry over to improved locomotor performance has not been demonstrated.
- **Different types of exercise.** No clear advantage has been demonstrated of adding isokinetic, resisted, or active exercise regimens to functional therapy alone (see Table 19).
- **Sensory retraining.** Chronic sensory deficits are often refractory and one recent study (see Table 19) found that sensory retraining improved performance on tests of impairment; however, the study did not examine measures of function (Yekutiel and Guttman, 1993).

Table 16. Evidence on the effectiveness of biofeedback

Author Year Country	Purpose Study design Duration of deficits Number of subjects	Outcome measures Maximum followup	Conclusions/ comments
Mandel, Nymark, Balmer, et al. (1990) Canada	Compare rhythmic positional BFB to EMG BFB RCT Chronic deficits N=37	Active ROM of ankle Dynamic dorsi- and plantarflexion Gait analysis Energy expenditure F/U until 3 months	Walking speed of both BFB groups improved more than controls, but differences significant only for positional BFB. Energy expenditure decreased in both BFB groups.
Wolf, LeCraw, and Barton (1989) United States	Compare effects of motor copy and conventional BFB RCT Chronic deficits N=26	Functional tasks Active ROM Integrated EMG levels F/U until 9 months	Significant functional improvements in both groups.
Basmajian, Gowland, Finlayson, et al. (1987) Canada	Compare integrated behavioral PT with BFB to traditional PT Mix of acute and chronic deficits N=29	UEFT Finger oscillation Health Belief Survey Mood and affect F/U until 9 months	No significant differences between groups. Both groups improved significantly on UEFT and finger oscillation.
John (1986) United Kingdom	Examine benefits of EMG BFB in the legs RCT with crossover at 3 weeks Acute deficits N=24	ROM Gait speed Static contraction F/U until 6 weeks	No significant differences in function.
Mulder, Hulstijn, and van der Meer (1986) Holland	Examine benefits of EMG BFB in the legs RCT Duration of deficits not available N=12	ROM Gait velocity	No differences among groups.

See notes at end of table.

Table 16. Evidence on the effectiveness of biofeedback (continued)

Author Year Country	Purpose Study design Duration of deficits Number of subjects	Outcome measures Maximum followup	Conclusions/ comments
Inglis, Donald, Monga, et al. (1984) Canada	Examine benefits of EMG BFB in the arm RCT with crossover of control group Deficits < 6 months N=30	Strength ROM Brunnstrom stages Post-test	No significant differences.
Basmajian, Gowland, Brandstater, et al. (1982) Canada	Compare effects of PT plus EMG BFB to PT alone RCT Deficits 2 to 5 months N=37	UEFT Post-test	No significant differences on any groups.
Burnside, Tobias, and Bursill (1982) United Kingdom	Compare BFB to exercise therapy for foot drop Non-RCT; matched control group Deficits > 3 months N=22	Strength ROM Gait (video) F/U until 6 weeks	BFB group improved significantly more on strength, ROM, and gait.
Greenberg and Fowler (1980) United States	Compare effects of kinetic BFB on elbow extension to OT alone RCT Chronic deficits N=20	Active elbow extension Post-test	No differences among groups.
Hurd, Pegram, and Nepomuceno (1980) United States	Compare EMG BFB to PT only and PT plus simulated BFB RCT Patients and muscles within patients randomly assigned Mean > 60 days N=44	Muscle activity Active ROM Post-test	Both BFB groups improved more than control "PT only" groups. No differences between BFB and simulated BFB groups.

See notes at end of table.

Table 16. Evidence on the effectiveness of biofeedback (continued)

Author Year Country	Purpose Study design Duration of deficits Number of subjects	Outcome measures Maximum followup	Conclusions/ comments
Shiavi, Champion, Freeman, et al. (1979) United States	Compare effects of EMG BFB in the leg to sham BFB and PT alone RCT Acute deficits N=22	Muscle control Manual muscle test	Results difficult to interpret.
Basmajian, Kukulka, Narayan, et al. (1975) United States	Compare effects on foot drop of BFB to PT alone RCT Deficits > 3 months N=20	Strength Active ROM Gait analysis F/U up to 16 weeks	Trends favor BFB but differences not significant.

Note: BFB = biofeedback. EMG = electromyographic. F/U = followup. OT = occupational therapy. PT = physical therapy. RCT = randomized controlled trial. ROM = range of motion. UEFT = Upper Extremity Function Test.

Table 17. Evidence on the effectiveness of functional electrical stimulation with or without biofeedback

Author Year Country	Purpose Study design Duration of deficits Number of subjects	Outcome measures Maximum followup	Conclusions/ comments
Kraft, Fitts, and Hammond (1992) United States	Compare two types of FES, proprioceptive PT, and no treatment in the arm Non-RCT with matched control groups Chronic deficits N=18	Fugl-Meyer Grip strength F/U up to 9 months	Results favor EMG stimulation group.
Levin and Hui-Chan (1992) Canada	Test effectiveness of transcutaneous electrical nerve stimulation (TENS) in chronic spasticity of lower extremities RCT with placebo control Chronic deficits N=13	Spasticity score Reflex profile Maximal contraction F/U at 3 weeks	Significant differences in outcomes favored TENS.
Cozean, Pease, and Hubbell (1988) United States	Compare the effects on gait of FES, BFB, and the combination RCT Mixed acute and chronic deficits N=36	Quantitative gait analysis (videos) F/U at 6 weeks	Results favor combined BFB and FES.
Winchester, Montgomery, Bowman, et al. (1983) United States	Compare effects of positional feedback plus FES to PT alone on knee extension RCT Deficit < 6 months N=40	Passive and active ROM Maximum isometric knee extension torque F/U at 4 weeks	Differences on knee extension torque favor BFB plus FES group.

See notes at end of table.

Table 17. Evidence on the effectiveness of functional electrical stimulation with or without biofeedback (continued)

Author Year Country	Purpose Study design Duration of deficits Number of subjects	Outcome measures Maximum followup	Conclusions/ comments
Bowman, Baker, and Waters (1979) United States	Compare effects on wrist extension of positional BFB and FES to PT alone RCT 3 weeks to 4 months N=30	Wrist extension torque Active ROM F/U at 4 weeks	Differences on both outcomes favor BFB plus FES group.
Merletti, Zelaschi, Latella, et al. (1978) Italy	Compare effects on ankle dorsiflexion of FES to PT alone RCT Deficits 1 to 15 months N=49	Maximum voluntary movement F/U at 4 weeks	Improvement greater in FES group ($p = 0.007$).
Takebe, Kukulka, Narayan, et al. (1976) United States	Compare effects of FES, PT plus BFB, and PT alone in spastic lower extremity Deficits > 3 months N=15	Gait analysis Ankle dorsiflexion ROM Post-test	Qualitative analysis favors BFB and FES groups.

Note: BFB = biofeedback. EMG = electromyographic. FES = functional electrical stimulation. F/U = followup. PT = physical therapy. RCT = randomized controlled trial. ROM = range of motion.

Table 18. Evidence on the effectiveness of treatment of disturbed balance

Author Year Country	Purpose Study design Duration of deficits Number of subjects	Outcome measures Maximum followup	Conclusions/ comments
Tangeman, Banaitis, and Williams (1990) United States	Test whether rehab improves balance and function Time series Chronic deficits N=40	Weight-shift balance ADL F/U until 3 months	Significant improvement on all measures that was sustained at 3 months.
Winstein, Gardner, McNeal, et al. (1989) United States	Compare effect of PT plus retraining to PT alone Non-RCT with matched control group Acute deficits N=42	Static center of pressure position Weight distribution Locomotor performance, gait pattern, coordination F/U at 3 to 4 weeks	Better standing symmetry in experimental group, but no differences in stability during locomotor performance.
Shumway-Cook, Anson, and Haller (1988) United States	Compare PT plus balance retraining and static force platform BFB to PT alone RCT Deficits < 6 months N=16	Lateral sway displacement Sway area F/U at 2 weeks	Lateral sway displacement reduced in experimental group, but no differences in total sway area.
Hocherman, Dickstein, and Pillar (1984) Israel	Compare PT plus platform training to PT alone Non-RCT with matched control group Acute deficits N=24	Maximal Movement Amplitude (MMA) Weight distribution F/U at 3 weeks	Experimental group improved stance stability and weight distribution more.

Note: ADL = activities of daily living. BFB = biofeedback. F/U = followup. PT = physical therapy. RCT = randomized controlled trial. Rehab = rehabilitation.

Table 19. Evidence on the effectiveness of other interventions to treat sensorimotor deficits

Author Year Country	Purpose Study design Duration of deficits Number of subjects	Outcome measures Maximum followup	Conclusions/ comments
Taub, Miller, Novack, et al. (1993) United States	Examine the effects of restraining the unaffected arm RCT Chronic deficits N=9	Emory Motor Function Test Arm Motor Activity Test (AMAT) Motor Activity Log Videotaped Motor Test F/U until 2 years	Restraint group improved more on multiple measures. Effects maintained at 2 years.
Yekutiel and Guttman (1993) Israel	Evaluate effects of sensory retraining Non-RCT with matched controls Chronic deficits N=39	Location of touch Elbow position 2-point discrimination Stereognosis F/U at 6 weeks	Significant differences favored sensory retraining group on all measures.
Wolf, LeCraw, Barton, et al. (1989) United States	Examine effects of "forced use" on the paretic arm Time series Chronic deficits N=21	21 timed activities 3 force measures F/U until 12 months	Forced use led to significant improvement in timed tasks. Effect maintained at 1 year.
Glasser (1986) United States	Compare effects on ambulation of PT plus isokinetic exercise to PT alone RCT Deficits 3 to 6 months N=20	Functional Ambulation Profile Ambulation time F/U at 5 weeks	No differences among groups.
Trombly, Thayer-Nason, Bliss, et al. (1986) United States	Compare different types of exercises on finger extension RCT Acute deficits N=20	ROM Tapping Grasp/release Daily pre- and post-tests	No significant differences among groups.

See notes at end of table.

Table 19. Evidence on the effectiveness of other interventions to treat sensorimotor deficits (continued)

Author Year Country	Purpose Study design Duration of deficits Number of subjects	Outcome measures Maximum followup	Conclusions/ comments
Inaba, Edberg, Montgomery, et al. (1973) United States	Compare functional training, active exercise, and restrictive exercise RCT Deficits < 4 months N=77	ADL Extension strength F/U until 2 months	No significant differences among groups at 2 months.

Note: ADL = activities of daily living. F/U = followup. PT = physical therapy. RCT = randomized controlled trial. ROM = range of motion.

Compensatory Techniques To Improve Functional Performance

Recommendation: Patients with persistent, nonremediable, functional deficits should be taught compensatory methods for performing important tasks and activities, using the affected limb when possible and, when not, the unaffected limb. (Research evidence=NA; expert opinion=strong consensus.)

Compensatory treatments address the tasks and activities that comprise meaningful roles for a person. Examples are:

- **Self-care tasks or basic ADL.** The ability to take care of basic personal needs including feeding, bathing, toileting, dressing, and grooming.
- **Complex tasks, or IADL.** The ability to perform more complex daily activities such as using the telephone, writing, cutting fingernails, driving a car, managing the home, and managing finances.
- **Social, recreational, and spiritual roles.** Examples are maintaining friendships, being an active parishioner, and pursuing valued hobbies.
- **Work.** The ability to engage in activities for financial remuneration.

Deficits that interfere with independence in these roles include:

- Inability to use an arm or hand to stabilize an object or perform an activity that requires the use of both arms or hands.
- Disturbed sensation or astereognosis (inability to perceive an object by feel alone), which prevents doing activities with tools or utensils out of the line of vision.
- Disturbed body scheme or spatial relationships which interfere with manipulating objects in the environment or in relation to one's own body. Unilateral neglect is particularly limiting because the person fails

to pay attention to anything in the neglected space and will, for example, eat only food on one side of the plate, shave only one side of the face, fail to dress one side of the body, and bump into objects on one side.

- Topographic agnosia, a perceptual impairment that limits independent mobility by preventing the person from finding the way from one place to another.
- Limited mobility, which interferes with turning over in bed, making transfers between bed and chair or toilet, or negotiating stairs.
- Communication problems that interfere with family relationships or are deterrents to the resumption of social and vocational roles.
- Alexia (inability to read) and agraphia (inability to write), which interfere with home management, financial management, some social roles, and work.
- Apraxia (inability to do purposeful movement that is not attributed to sensory or motor deficits), which can interfere with all tasks and activities, although the ability to do habitual tasks may be preserved enough in some patients to allow semi-independence in self care.
- Cognitive deficits that prevent the patient from understanding even one-step commands and preclude independence in most role functions.
- Incoordination or lack of dexterity in the nondominant hand when the dominant hand was the one affected by the stroke. This can severely limit independence. Practice and perseverance are needed to learn to use the nonaffected arm.
- Perceptual deficits and problems with motor learning, which have deleterious effects on the ability to perform tasks of daily living.

The objective of compensatory treatment is to help patients learn new skills that permit them to perform desired activities despite persisting motor, sensory, or cognitive deficits. Training begins with relatively simple tasks and progresses gradually to more difficult ones until the patient's limits are reached. Graduated challenges offer the opportunity for success and with it an increasing sense of competency, mastery, and self-esteem. Many adaptive methods aim to teach patients to perform tasks with one hand. Examples include ways to stabilize objects or clothing while working on them with the unimpaired arm or ways to fasten clothing with one hand.

Achievements are highly individual. Even patients who only have the ability to follow one-step commands and must use a wheelchair can achieve some independence in simple self-care tasks in a supportive environment. Without support, such patients are likely to require custodial care.

Most evidence supporting the effectiveness of compensatory techniques is indirect and depends on studies that show improvement in patient function during rehabilitation, but either do not test a particular technique or do not control for the effects of spontaneous neurological recovery.

Exceptions are controlled studies that have found short-term increases in walking speed in response to training regimens (Cozean, Pease, and Hubbell, 1988; Mandel, Nymark, Balmer, et al., 1990; Wade, Collen, Robb, et al., 1992).

Adaptive Devices, Durable Equipment, and Orthotic Devices

Recommendation: Adaptive devices should be used only if other methods of performing the task are not available or cannot be learned. The device should have proven reliability and safety, and the patient and/or caregiver should be thoroughly trained in its proper use. (Research evidence=NA; expert opinion=consensus.)

Many different types of adaptive devices and durable medical equipment are available to assist the patient in becoming more independent (examples are provided in Table 20). Need is determined by the type and level of the patient's functional deficit(s), the degree of adaptation achieved, and the structural characteristics of the living environment.

Use of a device should not substitute for reasonable efforts to teach a patient a method for performing the task in question. In most instances, mastery of the method will allow greater flexibility, satisfaction, and independence. The device may serve as a useful supplement, however, or permit a function to be performed if the adapted method cannot be learned or requires too much effort.

The patient and family/caregivers should be involved in the selection of adaptive devices and should be thoroughly trained in their use. Adequate attention to these matters will increase the likelihood that the device is wanted, is sufficient to meet needs, and will be fully used. Since some of these devices are expensive, the patient's financial circumstances and insurance coverage also need to be explored.

Recommendation: A wheelchair prescription for a patient with severe motor weakness or easy fatigability should be based on careful assessment of the patient and the environment in which the wheelchair will be used. Wheelchair selection should have the full support of the patient and family/involved others. (Research evidence=NA; expert opinion=strong consensus.)

Wheelchair designs vary widely and need to be adapted to the patient's special needs. Comfort, safety, proper posture, and access to home and community resources are important considerations. These objectives can be achieved only through careful assessment of both the patient and the environment, and through responsiveness to the wishes of patient and family.

Table 20. Examples of adaptive devices and durable equipment

Eating devices ■ Built-up handles on utensils for weak or incomplete grasp. ■ Rocker knife for one-handed cutting. ■ Nonskid mats to stabilize plate for eating with one hand. ■ Plate guards or scoop dishes for scooping food off the plate when eating one-handed. ■ Cups that hold liquid in the upper part and reduce the need to tilt the head when drinking, for patients with a swallowing problem who are at risk of aspiration.
Bathing and grooming devices ■ Long-handled sponge for limited reach. ■ Washcloth or sponge mitt for patients with a weak grasp. ■ Electric razors with specially adapted heads (e.g., at 90 degrees to the handle). ■ Hand-held shower nozzle. ■ Nonskid mats secured in tub or shower to prevent slipping and falling. ■ A wide selection of grab bars for use in tub or shower that require assessment of the patient's level of need, and the architectural limitations of the bathroom before selecting the design.
Toileting aids ■ Bedside commode, urinal, bedpan. ■ Elevated toilet seat. ■ Toilet seat with rails. ■ Grab bars next to the toilet.
Shower and tub aids ■ Shower and tub seats designed for decreased ability to stand in shower or sit down in or rise from the tub. ■ Shower and tub transfer seats for difficulty with shower and tub transfers and difficulty with standing in shower or sitting in tub. ■ Shower chairs that can be pushed into wheelchair-accessible shower for inability to transfer or stand while showering. ■ Hydraulic and motorized tub lifts if the patient is unable to get into or out of tub; use depends on architecture of bathroom.
Dressing equipment ■ Velcro closures for one-handed dressing. ■ Elasticized shoestrings for one-handed dressing. ■ Long-handled shoe horn when reach is limited.

Table 20. Examples of adaptive devices and durable equipment (continued)

Walking devices
■ Cane with a single point of contact that improves stability of gait when leg is weak. Cane should be fitted to the patient and have a rubber tip to improve traction. ■ Tripod or quad cane with three or four points of contact. These provide greater stability but are bulkier and more difficult to handle. ■ Folding cane chair, allowing the user to walk and then sit and rest. ■ Walkers that differ according to structure and purpose but must be lightweight and fold if the patient is to use them outside the home. ■ Adjustable pickup walkers for patients who need support to stand and walk, and are able to lift the walker and maintain balance. ■ Reciprocal walkers for patients who might lose their balance when lifting a regular walker. ■ Rolling walkers that increase energy-efficient walking, but may be too unstable for some patients.
Wheelchair and wheelchair cushions
■ Wheelchair. Wheelchair selection is based on body measurements, specific needs (e.g., elevating leg rests), safety, comfort, and maneuverability. A wheelchair for patients with hemiplegia may have a lowered base of support and lowered seat to permit the patient to use the uninvolved foot to propel the wheelchair or a one-armed drive that allows maneuvering with one arm and hand. ■ Wheelchair cushion. This is important for comfort and to prevent skin breakdown; selection is based on the patient's mobility status, body build, nutrition, and skin condition.
Transfer devices
■ Plastic or wooden transfer board to assist the patient who is unable to stand to perform bed, chair, shower, tub, or car sliding transfers. ■ Gait/transfer belt for use by caregiver, if indicated. ■ Hydraulic lifts for bed, chair, tub, or car transfers. ■ Hydraulic or electric stair lifts for patients unable to climb stairs. ■ Chairs modified to have higher seats for patients unable to lift out of seat. Electrically or mechanically powered chairs with seats that raise are available but are rarely indicated.
Leisure and recreation devices
■ Automatic card shufflers. ■ Card holders. ■ Large-faced cards. ■ Books on audio tape. ■ Swimming flotations. ■ Fishing pole harnesses. ■ Gardening tools with builtup handles. ■ Specially designed golf clubs.

Recommendation: Lower extremity orthotic devices should be considered if ankle or knee stabilization is needed to help the patient walk. Prefabricated bracing can be used initially, and more expensive customized bracing reserved for patients who demonstrate a long-term need. (Research evidence=NA; expert opinion=consensus.)

Timely use of orthotic devices can facilitate ambulation, permit gait training to be conducted simultaneously with muscle control exercises, and reduce the energy cost of ambulation in the presence of hemiparesis (Corcoran, Jebsen, Brengelmann, et al., 1970). Use of orthotic devices should not, however, be substituted for functional exercise directed at improving muscle strength and control, if the prognosis for recovery of motor control is good.

Preventing and Treating Complications

Prevention of complications such as aspiration pneumonia, dehydration or malnutrition, skin breakdown, urinary tract infections, and falls was discussed in Chapter 4. This section addresses the prevention of falls in a rehabilitation setting and the prevention and treatment of muscle spasticity and contracture, shoulder injuries, and pain syndromes.

Fall Prevention

Recommendation: The patient's risk of falling should be evaluated on admission to a rehabilitation program, and preventive measures should be taken that are appropriate to the patient's deficits. (Research evidence=NA; expert opinion=strong consensus.)

Patients with strokes have 61 to 83 percent of all falls that occur in rehabilitation hospitals (DeVincenzo and Watkins, 1987; Mion, Gregor, Chwirchak, et al., 1989). Many of the same considerations concerning fall prevention apply as discussed previously in Chapter 4. The major difference is that the patient's risk of falling is increased by rehabilitation treatments aimed at increasing mobility. Safety measures need to anticipate these risks and ensure environmental precautions and adequate supervision.

Muscle weakness, problems with gait or balance, difficulties with transfers, altered sensation, postural hypotension, impaired vision, and confusion or disorientation each increase the risk of falls. Falls are particularly likely when the patient tries to reach the toilet without assistance. Acute illnesses, generalized weakness, and drug side effects compound risks due to neurological deficits. Patients with visual neglect who are slow in performing tasks are at high risk of multiple accidents (Diller and Weinberg, 1970); and wheelchair users with visuospatial deficits are at increased risk of running into obstacles (Webster, Rapport, Godlewski, et al., 1994). Behavioral impulsivity, older age, a history of previous falls, and multiple transfers are associated with an increased risk of falling (Rapport, Webster, Fleming, et al., 1993). Equally important as injuries from falls is the possibility that fear of falling may compromise a patient's confidence and reduce motivation to walk or attempt self-care activities.

Facilitywide fall prevention programs need to address environmental hazards such as accessibility of toileting facilities, inadequate lighting, and wet and slippery floors. Patient risk profiles for falling should be updated at regular intervals to reflect changes in functional status and activity level. Timely assistance to satisfy bathroom needs, adequate supervision during rehabilitation sessions and intervening periods of practice, and patient and family education in fall prevention strategies are all important. Medication regimens should be adjusted to avoid sedation, confusion, or postural hypotension. Technologic approaches such as antitipping devices on wheelchairs, bed and chair alarm systems, wedge seat cushions, and—as a last resort—use of restraints are helpful in some patients.

Despite preventive measures, falls do sometimes occur. It is important that patients be taught how to get up after a fall and that family members be taught how to evaluate the possibility of a fracture, and if a fracture has not occurred, to help the patient get up. Most falls can be managed without outside assistance.

Spasticity and Contractures

Recommendation: Spasticity and contractures should be treated/ prevented by antispastic pattern positioning, range-of-motion exercises, stretching and/or splinting. (Research evidence=NA; expert opinion=consensus.)

Contractures that restrict movement of the involved joint or are painful will impede rehabilitation and may limit the patient's potential for recovery. Paretic limbs with muscle spasticity are at especially high risk of developing contracture. Prevention is the key to effective management. Traditional measures are to support the limb in an anatomically correct position that opposes the usual pattern of spasticity, and to move it through its full ranges of motion at regular intervals. The limited evidence from controlled trials of treatments for spasticity in patients with strokes is summarized in Table 21. Manual stretch may be effective with selected patients (Carey, 1990). The use of medications to treat spasticity is controversial. For example, one randomized trial found that dantrolene sodium had no effect on the spastic limb but decreased strength in the unaffected limb (Katrak, Cole, Poulos, et al., 1992).

If a contracture interferes with function, corrective measures include splinting or casting involved joints into progressively more anatomically correct positions and surgical corrections. One study that used inflatable splints in the arm was inconclusive (Poole, Whitney, Hangeland, et al., 1990). Motor-point nerve blocks using phenol or botulinum toxin may

Table 21. Evidence on the effectiveness of treatment for spasticity

Author Year Country	Purpose Study design Duration of deficits Number of subjects	Outcome measures Maximum followup	Conclusions/ comments
Katrak, Cole, Poulos, et al. (1992) Australia	Examine effects of dantrolene sodium on spasticity and muscle strength Double-blinded RCT with crossover Acute deficits N=31	Motor Assessment Scale (MAS) Cybex isokinetic dynamometer ADL (Barthel) F/U until 13 weeks	Dantrolene sodium decreased strength in unaffected limbs but had no effect in impaired limbs.
Carey (1990) United States	Examine effects of manual stretch on finger control RCT Chronic deficits N=24	EMG ratios of flexor and extensor muscles Joint Movement Tracking Test (JMTT) Force Tracking Test (FTT) Immediate post-test	Stretch group improved more than stroke controls on JMTT but not on FTT.
Poole, Whitney, Hangeland, et al. (1990) United States	Test effects of inflatable pressure splints on upper extremity function RCT with matched pairs design Duration of deficits not available N=18	Fugl-Meyer F/U at 3 weeks	No significant differences.

Note: ADL = activities of daily living. EMG = electromyographic. F/U = followup. RCT = randomized controlled trial.

have roles in selected patients (Awad and Dykstra, 1990), but their effectiveness in stroke has not been studied in controlled trials.

Shoulder Injury and Pain Syndromes

The patient with a stroke may experience pain from arthritis, peripheral vascular disease, or osteoporosis; may develop pain from muscle spasms or soft tissue or joint injury in a paretic limb; or may experience specific types of pain syndromes such as reflex sympathetic dystrophy or the thalamic pain syndrome.

Recommendation: The prevention of shoulder injuries should emphasize proper positioning and support and avoidance of overly vigorous range-of-motion exercises. (Research evidence=C; expert opinion=strong consensus.)

Some degree of shoulder pain has been reported in as many as 70 to 84 percent of patients with a paralyzed upper extremity (Brandstater and Basmajian, 1987; Roy, 1988) but is severe in oniy a small percentage of patients. The shoulder is especially vulnerable to injury because the joint capsule depends on the surrounding muscle cuff for support. Flaccid paralysis permits gravitational pull to stretch the joint capsule. Prolonged pain, "frozen" shoulder, and decreased functional independence are potential results of shoulder injury.

Prevention, first and foremost, requires awareness of susceptibility to shoulder injury. Preventive measures include supporting the shoulder in a position that maintains a normal scapulo-humoral orientation, using lap trays on wheelchairs, using a pull sheet rather than lifting under the arms to pull the patient up in bed, and maintaining proper positioning and support in bed and while sitting or standing. Range-of-motion exercises should not carry the shoulder beyond 90 degrees of flexion and abduction unless there is upward rotation of the scapula and external rotation of the humeral head. Patients who are taught self-range of motion should be cautioned to avoid excessive shoulder flexion. Use of an overhead pulley appears to increase the frequency of pain (Kumar, Metter, Mehta, et al., 1990). The use of slings or arm supports is controversial because of the potential complications from immobilization.

Reflex sympathetic dystrophy (RSD), which has been reported in 12 to 25 percent of patients with hemiplegia (Brandstater and Basmajian, 1987), is characterized by pain, swelling, stiffness, and discoloration of the involved limb and shoulder. Its cause is not fully understood, but immobility, venous pooling, altered muscle tone, and inflammation of the shoulder joint appear to contribute. Treatment of RSD involves graded and carefully selected range-of-motion exercises, heat, compression, high-dose anti-inflammatory agents, pulse steroid therapy, pain medications, sympathetic nerve blocks, and therapeutic positioning (Borgman and Passarella,1991; Brandstater and Basmajian, 1987; Johnston and Olson, 1980).

Managing Cognitive and Perceptual Deficits

Recommendation: Cognitive deficits that preclude effective learning are contraindications to rehabilitation. Cognitive and perceptual problems not severe enough to preclude rehabilitation require goal-directed treatment plans. (Research evidence=NA; expert opinion=strong consensus.)

Knowledge of the patient's cognitive and perceptual limitations is important in planning and conducting the rehabilitation regimen, helping to prepare the patient for functioning safely after the return home, and predicting the ability to resume vocational activities.

Cognitive deficits may involve problems with attention, orientation, concentration, learning (short-term memory), or problem solving. Common specific patterns are unilateral neglect (or hemi-inattention) and apraxia. Unilateral neglect is a disturbance of a patient's awareness of space on the side of the body opposite the location of the stroke-causing lesion. Apraxia is a disorder of learned movement that cannot be explained by the patient's deficits in strength, coordination, sensation, or comprehension.

Diffuse cognitive deficits occur more frequently in patients with large frontal strokes, visuospatial deficits in right hemisphere strokes, and apraxia in left hemisphere strokes. The true frequency of these deficits is obscured by their diverse manifestations and by the use of varying diagnostic criteria (Schenkenberg, Bradford, and Ajax, 1980; Wilson, Cockburn, and Halligan, 1987). In the Framingham Study cohort, cognitive performance was found to be significantly lower 6 months after a stroke than before the event (Kase, Wolf, Kelly-Hayes, et al., 1987). Cognitive disturbances tend to improve after a stroke but may persist for months or years. One population-based study found that 29 percent of patients still had problems with memory 3 months after returning to the community (Wade, Parker, and Langton-Hewer, 1986). Unilateral neglect has been reported in as many as half of patients with right brain damage and in 20 to 25 percent of patients with left brain damage 3 months after the onset of stroke (Fullerton, McSherry, and Stout, 1986; Stone, Wilson, Wroot, et al., 1991), but estimates of incidence vary due to differences in the populations studied, time since onset of stroke, and the assessment measures used.

Perceptual problems impede performance of many activities of daily living (Ben-Yishay, Gerstman, Diller, et al., 1970; Denes, Semenza, Stoppa, et al., 1982; Kinsella and Ford, 1980; Wade, Wood, and Hewer, 1988). Patients with spatial·constructional problems have difficulty dressing, eating, walking, and grooming (Warren, 1990), and those with unilateral neglect experience difficulty in academic tasks (reading, writing, arithmetic), grooming, reading a menu, using a telephone, and driving an automobile (Gordon and Diller, 1983; Titus, Gall, Yerxa, et al., 1991). Effects on task performance depend on the pattern of cognitive deficits. For example, patients with left hemiparesis often experience accidents that are related to difficulties in dealing with space, while accidents in patients with right hemiparesis are often related to slowness in processing information (Diller and Weinberg, 1970).

Unawareness of the stroke (or its manifestations) is often found in patients with lesions in the nondominant hemisphere. It can lead to impulsive, unsafe behavior in a patient who may otherwise appear relatively normal with respect to physical functioning. In general, the degree of unawareness is related to the extent of brain damage (Levine,

1990) and the degree of cognitive impairment (Diller and Weinberg, 1993). Flagrant denial is usually found in patients with severe mental confusion who are unlikely to be admitted to rehabilitation programs. Denial of specific impairments or areas of disability is common, however, and poses special challenges. In general, patients are more aware of motor impairments than of cognitive impairments or emotional problems (Anderson and Tranel, 1989; Hibbard, Gordon, Stein, et al., 1992). There are no standard approaches to managing unawareness. The therapist needs to characterize its dimensions and develop strategies to minimize its effects (Levine, 1990).

The presence of cognitive or perceptual deficits often increases the severity of functional disabilities, causes emotional distress, interferes with the patient's ability to participate in and learn during rehabilitation, and increases the risk of injury. Cognitive and perceptual deficits may also interfere with personal, family, and environmental adaptation after the return home, and require special efforts to prepare the patient and family for transition.

Treatments for cognitive and perceptual deficits emphasize retraining, substitution of intact abilities, and compensatory approaches. Goals are to remediate the impairment or to reduce the impact of the deficit through repetitive exercises or compensatory treatments that teach patients new methods of response. Evidence of the effectiveness of these techniques (see Table 22) is limited to short-term effects on outcome measures that share stimulus characteristics with the intervention (Carter, Caruso, Languirand, et al., 1980; Gordon, Hibbard, Egelko, et al., 1985; Soderback, 1988). Several studies have demonstrated the ability to train patients to improve their visual scanning skills, somatosensory awareness, and visual perception skills; however, no study has demonstrated that these skills persist or carry over to functional activities (Gordon, Hibbard, Egelko, et al., 1985; Weinberg, Diller, Gordon, et al., 1977 and 1979; Weinberg, Piasetsky, Diller, et al., 1982). Case studies that have combined skill training with training in a functional activity are inconclusive. Strategies that have been tried for treating neglect include caloric stimulation (Rubens, 1985), Fresnel prisms (Rossi, Kheyfets, and Reding, 1990), eye-patching (Butter and Kirsh, 1992), dynamic stimulation (Butter, Kirsch, and Reeves, 1990), and optokinetic stimulation (Pizzamiglio, Frasca, Guariglia, et al., 1990); however, there is no evidence of lasting benefits from these.

The goal of treatment for apraxia is to restore the person's ability to perform appropriate habitual or novel movements. Treatments include manually guided movement, graded use of objects and contexts that evoke automatic motor responses, mental imagery, and backward chaining. However, evidence supporting the effectiveness of these treatments is limited.

Table 22. Evidence on the effectiveness of treatment for cognitive and perceptual deficits

Author Year Country	Purpose Study design Duration of deficits Number of subjects	Outcome measures Maximum followup	Conclusions/ comments
Robertson, Gray, Pentland, et al. (1990) United Kingdom	Test effectiveness of microcomputer programs for unilateral visual field neglect "Semi-RCT" with randomized blocks of severely and mildly affected patients Group means of 11 and 19 weeks N=36	Behavior Inattention Test (BIT) Psychometric battery F/U until 6 months	No significant differences among groups.
Rossi, Kheyfets, and Reding (1990) United States	Test effects of Fresnel prisms in homonymous hemianopsia or visual neglect RCT Acute deficits N=39	Battery of visual perception tests ADL (Barthel) Number of falls F/U until 4 weeks	Prisms improved scores on visual perception tests ($p < 0.01$), but differences not significant for ADL or falls.
Soderback (1988) Sweden	Test effects of intellectual function and intellectual housework training RCT Group means of 60 and 81 days N=70	Intellectual Function Assessment (IFA) Intellectual Housework Assessment (IHA) Psychometric battery F/U until 6 months	Initial benefits of training on IHA measures not sustained at 6 months.
Gordon, Hibbard, Egelko, et al. (1985) United States	Test effects of specific training protocols in visual perceptive disorders "Quasi-RCT" (alternate wards) Acute deficits > 4 weeks N=77	Extensive test battery F/U until 4 months	Experimental group improved more on specifically trained skills, but differences not sustained.

See notes at end of table.

Table 22. Evidence on the effectiveness of treatment for cognitive and perceptual deficits (continued)

Author Year Country	Purpose Study design Duration of deficits Number of subjects	Outcome measures Maximum followup	Conclusions/ comments
Carter, Howard, and O'Neil (1983) United States	Test effects of cognitive skill remediation RCT Acute deficits N=33	Visual scanning Visuospatial matching to sample Time estimation Post-test	Significant differences on all measures.
Carter,Caruso, Languirand, et al. (1980) United States	Test effects of cognitive skill remediation RCT Acute deficits N=37	Letter cancellation Visuospatial matching Digit span Verbal-free recall Time estimation Post-test	Experimental group improved more on letter cancellation and visuospatial matching. Results based on only 18 of 27 randomized patients.
Weinberg, Diller, Gordon, et al. (1979) United States	Test effects of visual scanning, spatial organization, and sensory awareness training in patients with right brain damage RCT Deficits > 4 weeks N=53	Psychological test battery (26 scores on 17 tests) F/U at 4 weeks	Experimental group improved significantly more on multiple tests. Effects greater in more severely impaired patients.
Weinberg, Diller, Gordon, et al. (1977) United States	Test effects of visual scanning training in patients with right brain damage RCT Deficits > 4 weeks N=57	Test battery (14 tests) F/U at 4 weeks	Significant differences on multiple tests.
Taylor, Schaeffer, Blumenthal, et al. (1971) United States	Test effects of perceptual training in patients with right brain damage RCT Deficits < 6 months N=78	Percept-Concept-Motor Function (PCMF) ADL Brunnstrom stages Social service interview Post-test	No differences among groups.

Note: ADL = activities of daily living. F/U = followup. RCT = randomized controlled trial.

Managing Emotional Disorders

Diagnosing and Treating Depression

Recommendation: A high index of suspicion needs to be maintained and appropriate steps should be taken to determine the presence and cause of depression. The diagnosis of depression depends primarily on the clinical examination, supplemented when necessary by the use of selected depression scales. (Research evidence=A; expert opinion=strong consensus.)

Depression is common after stroke, either as a direct biologic effect of the brain damage or as a reaction to disabling illness, and has been reported in 11 to 68 percent of patients, including major depression in 10 to 27 percent of patients (Eastwood, Rifat, Nobbs, et al., 1989; Ebrahim, Barer, and Nouri, 1987; Gordon, 1992; House, Dennis, Morgridge, et al., 1991; Morris, Robinson, and Raphael, 1990; Robinson and Benson, 1981; Robinson, Starr, Kubos, et al., 1983; Robinson and Szetela, 1981; Wade, Legh-Smith, and Hewer, 1987). Estimates vary with the diagnostic criteria used (Gordon, 1992). The time since stroke onset is also a factor, since depression tends to develop over time and is more likely to be diagnosed as rehabilitation proceeds than during the acute hospitalization or at the time of the baseline evaluation.

Depression in stroke can have many etiologies. These include (1) a normal reaction to the losses caused by a stroke, (2) an exacerbation of preexisting depressive personality features, (3) a specific psychiatric disorder such as major depression, (4) a medical condition (e.g., hypothyroidism or Addison's disease), (5) a medication (sedatives, antihypertensives), or (6) organic brain damage. Depression can produce cognitive deficits including problems with orientation, language, visual construction, motor function, and frontal lobe tasks (Bolla-Wilson, Robinson, Starkstein, et al., 1989), especially after left hemisphere injury (Downhill and Robinson, 1994; House, Dennis, Warlow, et al., 1990). Major depression has been linked to infarcts in the left anterior cerebral cortex and basal ganglia, minor depression to right-side posterior lesions and apathy, and paradoxical cheerfulness to right anterior lesions (Robinson and Benson, 1981; Robinson and Szetela, 1981). Often, depression in stroke is associated with more than one etiology. Only a weak relationship has been shown between the severity of depression and the severity of motor or cognitive impairment after stroke (Depression Guideline Panel, 1993 [sponsored by AHCPR]).

A diagnosis of depression should be considered when the patient persistently appears depressed; gives evidence of diminished interest in activities, loss of energy, loss of appetite, sleep disturbances, or an agitated state; or expresses feelings of worthlessness, impaired concentration, or suicidal thoughts. Changes from pre-stroke behaviors observed by family members and a history of previous depression may provide valuable clues.

A clinical interview by a knowledgeable mental health professional is the most effective method of diagnosis (assessment is discussed in Chapter 3).

Recommendation: The choice of treatment for depression will depend on the cause and the severity of symptoms. (Research evidence=C; expert opinion=consensus.)

Depression may adversely affect both participation in rehabilitation and long-term outcomes and may compound cognitive dysfunction (Bolla-Wilson, Robinson, Starkstein, et al., 1989). Documented effects include a higher 10-year mortality than that of nondepressed patients (Morris, Robinson, Andrzejewski, et al., 1993), longer lengths of stay in inpatient rehabilitation programs (Schubert, Burns, Paras, et al., 1992b), greater disability in ADL (Parikh, Robinson, Lipsey, et al., 1990; Schubert, Taylor, Lee, et al., 1992a), higher rates of discharge to an institution (Cushman, 1988), and lower levels of social activities (Gordon, Hibbard, Egelko, et al., 1985) and sexual functioning (Monga, Lawson, and Inglis, 1986). Fortunately, symptoms tend to resolve spontaneously during recovery; however, they may last for 2 years or more (Morris, Robinson, and Raphael, 1990; Robinson, Bolduc, and Price, 1987).

Effective treatment depends on an accurate diagnosis. The first step is to ensure that the patient is receiving the best possible care for other disabilities and that depressive symptoms are not due to medications (e.g., sedatives) or environmental factors (e.g., interruption of sleep habits or dissatisfaction with rehabilitation). Mild symptoms of depression will often respond to greater attention and encouragement from staff or family, simple changes in the environment, or active participation in therapeutic activities. More severe depression may respond to antidepressant medications or psychotherapy (cognitive, interpersonal, or behavioral). No controlled studies have examined the effectiveness of psychotherapy specifically in patients with depression due to stroke. The effectiveness of medications has been demonstrated in three small randomized controlled trials and is supported by numerous uncontrolled studies (Andersen, Verstergaard, and Lauritzen, 1994; Lipsey, Robinson, Pearlson, et al., 1984; Reding, Orto, Winter, et al., 1986). (For more information, see Table 23.)

Side effects from antidepressant medications are common in patients with strokes. When medications are used, drugs with favorable side-effect profiles are preferable. Alternatives include serotonin reuptake inhibitors and tricyclic antidepressants. Initial doses should be small and side effects should be closely monitored. Patients with major depression usually require treatment with medication. Regardless of which treatment modality is chosen, the patient's response should be assessed and treatments adjusted accordingly.

Evidence supporting methods of diagnosing and treating depression has been well documented in the literature and is summarized in an AHCPR-

Table 23. Evidence on the effectiveness of drug treatment of post-stroke depression

Author Year Country	Purpose Study design Duration of deficits Number of subjects	Outcome measures Maximum followup	Conclusions/ comments
Reding, Orto, Winter, et al. (1986) United States	Examine effectiveness of trazodone in post-stroke depression Triple-blinded RCT Acute deficits N=27	ADL (Barthel) F/U at 4 to 5 weeks	Treated group improved more, but results significant only for patients with a positive dexamethasone suppression test.
Lipsey, Robinson, Pearlson, et al. (1984) United States	Examine effectiveness of nortriptyline in post-stroke depression Double-blinded RCT Acute deficits N=34	Hamilton Depression Studies (HDS) Zung Depression Scale (ZDS) Present State Examination (PSE) Mini-Mental State (MMS) John Hopkins Functioning Inventory (JHFI) Social Ties Checklist (STC) F/U at 6 weeks	Treated group improved more on depression scales but not in functional abilities.

Note: ADL = activities of daily living. F/U = followup. RCT = randomized controlled trial.

sponsored guideline on depression (Depression Guideline Panel, 1993) and in a review article (Starkstein and Robinson, 1994).

Other Emotional Reactions to Stroke

Emotional disturbances such as apathy, mania, delusions, hallucinations, personality changes, and obsessive-compulsive disorders occur in patients with strokes (but are relatively rare). Emotional responses such as grief or anger over the losses of function due to stroke, anxiety, altered body image and self-esteem, emotional lability, and impulsive behaviors are more common. Diagnosis depends primarily on the clinical interview. Recognition of these problems is important so that precautions can be taken to protect patient safety, and treatment with behavioral approaches or medications can be given. The effectiveness of treatment has been well demonstrated for pathologic laughing and crying after stroke (Robinson, Parikh, Lipsey, et al., 1993).

Treating Speech and Language Disorders

Introduction

Speech or language disorders occur in as many as 40 percent of patients with strokes. Rapid spontaneous improvement is common; however, persisting problems may have pervasive consequences for the quality of a person's life, ranging from loss of employability to feelings of social isolation. Reactive depression, withdrawal, disruption of family roles, and loss of income are common.

Assessment of speech and language function is discussed in Chapter 3. Accurate documentation of deficits is required to guide the choice of treatments. For this reason, all patients with speech and language disorders should have a hearing evaluation, and the use of standardized tests (see Attachment 9) is strongly recommended.

Aphasia

Recommendation: Patients with aphasia should be offered treatment targeted at the identified language retrieval or comprehension deficits and aimed at improving functional communication. (Research evidence=C; expert opinion=consensus.)

Goals of treatment for aphasia are to (1) reinstate (remediate) the aphasic patient's ability to speak, comprehend, read, and write; (2) assist the patient in developing strategies that compensate for or circumvent language problems; (3) address associated psychological problems that compromise the quality of life of aphasic patients and their families; and (4) help the family and involved others to communicate with the patient.

A large number of techniques are used by speech-language pathologists. The following interventions have been studied experimentally or have been developed and tested in at least one treatment or treatment comparison study.

- Traditional stimulus-response modality-specific treatments and drills such as Language Oriented Treatment (LOT) (Shewan and Bandur, 1982), direct stimulus-response treatment (Wertz, Collins, Weiss, et al., 1981; Wertz, Weiss, Aten, et al., 1986), and Melodic Intonation Therapy (Therapeutics and Technology Assessment Subcommittee of the American Academy of Neurology, 1994).
- Methods that work on deficits that underlie language disorders such as perseveration and difficulties in symbol use, including Treatment of Aphasic Perseveration (TAP) (Helm-Estabrooks, Emery, and Albert, 1987) and Visual Action Therapy (VAT) (Helm-Estabrooks, Fitzpatrick, and Barresi, 1982).
- Methods that teach compensatory strategies designed to circumvent language deficits, such as Conversational Coaching (Holland, 1980) and

Promoting Aphasic Communicative Effectiveness (Davis and Wilcox, 1985).

- Methods that teach alternative and augmentative communication systems to aphasic adults. The best example is C-Vic (Weinrich, Steele, Carlson, et al., 1989).
- Developmental methods that represent attempts to apply emerging concepts from cognitive neuropsychology to the remediation of aphasia (Byng, 1988; Mitchum, Handiges, and Berndt, 1993).
- Programmatic approaches that combine features of all of the above. An illustration is furnished by Springer, Glindemann, and Huber (1991).

Treatment for aphasia can be integrated with treatments for sensorimotor or cognitive deficits or can be provided separately. Treatment should involve family and caregivers so that effective communication can be reestablished, and family members can be instructed in communication techniques.

Evidence from controlled trials on the effectiveness of treatment for aphasia is not conclusive (see Table 24). Some studies indicate benefit (Wertz, Collins, Weiss, et al., 1981; Wertz, Weiss, Aten, et al., 1986), while other studies fail to document sustained benefits (Hartman and Landau, 1987; Lincoln, McGuirk, Mulley, et al., 1984). To date, no study has examined the relationship between treatment effectiveness and the characteristics of the patient or tested the benefits of treatments specifically tailored to the patient's deficits. Treatment by trained volunteers appears to be equally effective as that by speech and language professionals, and results appear to be unaffected by delaying treatment (Wertz, Weiss, Aten, et al., 1986).

Right Hemisphere Communication Disorders

Goals of treatment for right hemisphere communication disorders are to increase awareness of deficits, reinstate communicative behaviors that have been disrupted, and provide compensatory techniques when restoration is not possible. Treatments are directed at the organization of language, its use in context, learning to interpret figurative language, and learning to use language in problem solving. Because right hemisphere language disorders are complex and their treatment is a relatively new field, the effectiveness of treatment has not been fully evaluated.

Dysarthria and Apraxia of Speech

Goals of treatment for dysarthria and apraxia of speech are to reinstate normal intelligibility to the dysarthric or apraxic person's speech or to use compensatory strategies or devices when intelligibility remains limited. Apraxia of speech, dysarthria, and aphasia often coexist. In such cases, the goal is to determine the contribution of each type of deficit to problems in functional communication and to develop an integrated treatment plan.

Table 24. Evidence on the effectiveness of treatment of speech and language deficits

Author Year Country	Purpose Study design Duration of deficits Number of subjects	Outcome measures Maximum followup	Conclusions/ comments
Poeck, Huber, and Willmes (1989) West Germany	Compare intense language treatment to spontaneous recovery and examine benefits of treatment 12 months post-stroke Non-RCT (unselected retrospective control group) Acute and chronic deficits N=229	Aachen Aphasia Test 8 week post-test	Differences significant in patients treated < 4 months after strokes, but not in patients treated later. 68% of chronic patients (> 12 months after stroke) improved significantly.
Hartman and Landau (1987) United States	Compare traditional language therapy to supportive counseling RCT Acute deficits N=60	PICA change score F/U until 10 months post-stroke	No significant differences between treatment groups.
Wertz, Weiss, Aten, et al. (1986) United States	Compare treatment to no treatment and treatment by speech and language professionals to trained volunteers; examine effects of delaying treatment RCT Acute deficits N=121	PICA scores F/U until 24 weeks	Differences between treatment and no treatment groups were significant, but not those between home treatment and no treatment, home treatment and clinic treatment, or earlier and deferred treatment.

See notes at end of table.

Table 24. Evidence on the effectiveness of treatment of speech and language deficits (continued)

Author Year Country	Purpose Study design Duration of deficits Number of subjects	Outcome measures Maximum followup	Conclusions/ comments
Lincoln, McGuirk, Mulley, et al. (1984) United Kingdom	Compare speech treatment to natural recovery RCT, but analysis confined to patients who completed 24 weeks of treatment and matched controls Acute deficits N=191 (327 randomized, but only 191 completed analysis)	PICA Functional Communication Profile F/U to 34 weeks post-stroke	No significant differences among groups. Only 27 subjects received > 36 treatment sessions.
Shewan and Kertesz (1984) N/A	Compare treatment by speech-language pathologists (SLPs) to treatment by trained volunteers; compare treatment to no treatment Partial RCT—random assignment to treatment groups; self-selected control group Acute deficits N=100	Western Aphasia Battery Auditory Comprehension Test for Sentences F/U until 1 year	Significantly greater improvement in treated group than (noncomparable) controls. No significant differences between treatment by SLP and trained volunteers or between language-oriented treatment and stimulus-facilitation treatment by SLP.
Wertz, Collins, Weiss, et al. (1981) United States	Compare individual with group treatment RCT Acute deficits N=67	PICA scores Token Test Word Fluency Test Colored Progressive Matrices Informant's rating Conversational rating F/U until 44 weeks	Significant differences favored individual for some PICA subtests but not other outcome measures.

See notes at end of table.

Table 24. Evidence on the effectiveness of treatment of speech and language deficits (continued)

Author Year Country	Purpose Study design Duration of deficits Number of subjects	Outcome measures Maximum followup	Conclusions/ comments
Basso, Capitani, and Vignolo (1979) N/A	Compare treatment to spontaneous recovery Non-RCT Mixed acute and chronic deficits N=281	Standard language exam F/U until 6 months	Treated patients improved more. Increased time post-onset and aphasia severity negatively associated with improvement.
Butfield and Zangwill (1946) N/A	Examine treatment outcomes Observational study Mixed acute and chronic deficits N=65	Clinical staff opinion, testing, and clinical records Varied F/U	Patients with less severe aphasia improved more. 78% of subjects improved with treatment. Study primarily of historic interest.

Note: F/U = followup. N/A = not available. PICA = Porch Index of Communicative Abilities. RCT = randomized controlled trial.

For dysarthric speakers, indirect treatment methods include sensory stimulation, exercises intended to strengthen speech musculature or modify muscle tone, modifying positioning and posture for speech, and improving respiratory capacity and efficiency. Direct methods include helping dysarthric speakers to produce speech under carefully arranged and controlled conditions. Because speech production typically encompasses respiration, phonation, resonation, articulation, and prosody, each may be the target of direct manipulation and modification.

Treatment for apraxia of speech focuses on the articulatory aspect of speech production. Emphasis is on relearning articulatory patterns and sequences of gestures, often hierarchically arranged to begin at relatively automatic levels and progress to more purposive communication. Intra- and intersystemic reorganization of the speech act is a programmatic approach based on learning to intone speech that has been used successfully in apractic speakers (Rosenbek, 1985; Wertz, 1984). Evidence supporting the effectiveness of treatments for dysarthria and apraxia of speech are limited to single-subject studies and case series.

Severely impaired dysarthric and apraxic speakers may benefit from alternative forms of communication or augmentative devices such as communication boards and books, pacing boards, and sophisticated electronic communication devices.

Discharge

Indications for Discharge

Recommendation: Discharge from a rehabilitation program should occur when reasonable treatment goals have been achieved. Absence of progress on two successive evaluations should lead to reconsideration of the treatment regimen or the appropriateness of the current setting. (Research evidence=NA; expert opinion=consensus.)

The term "reasonable treatment goals" is used to emphasize the importance of not underestimating or overestimating the patient's capabilities. When reasonable goals have been achieved, the patient is better served by moving to the next stage of recovery.

Lack of objective evidence of progress at two successive evaluations (i.e., over a period of 2 weeks in an intense program and 4 weeks in a less intense program) often indicates that a functional *ceiling* has been reached. Unless there is a good reason for the plateau in functional gain, transfer to a different level of care may be in the patient's best interests, and may also represent cost-effective use of rehabilitation resources.

Assessment Prior to Discharge

Recommendation: Assessment prior to discharge should include the patient's functional status, the proposed living environment, the adequacy of support by family or involved others, financial resources, and the availability of social and community supports. (Research evidence=NA; expert opinion=strong consensus.)

The predischarge assessment provides essential information for discharge planning, both about the patient and about the environment to which the patient will return. The assessment also provides a summary measure of gains achieved during the rehabilitation program and a baseline for monitoring subsequent progress. Performance of both basic and instrumental ADL is an important component of the assessment.

Discharge Planning

Overview

Recommendation: Discharge planning should begin at the time of admission; should be a systematic, interdisciplinary process, coordinated by a single health provider; should intimately involve the patient and family; and should include assessment of the patient's living environment, family/caregiver support, disability entitlements, and potential for vocational rehabilitation. To the maximum extent possible, all decisions should reflect a consensus among the patient,

family/caregivers, and rehabilitation team. (Research evidence=NA; expert opinion=strong consensus.)

Discharge from a rehabilitation program marks a critical point on the trajectory of post-stroke recovery and an important transition to new challenges. Discharge planning should begin on the day of admission to a rehabilitation program. At this time, initial information is obtained on the extent of family or caregiver support available and the potential places of residence after rehabilitation (in the case of inpatient programs). Goals of discharge planning are to:

- Identify a safe place of residence.
- Ensure that the patient and family/caregiver are adequately trained in essential skills.
- Arrange for continued medical care.
- Arrange for continued rehabilitation services.
- Arrange for needed community services.

Recommending a Safe Place of Residence. The main considerations in selecting a place of residence are the patient's disabilities, a realistic assessment of the family/caregiver's capabilities, and safety (all in the context of patient and family preferences). Safety refers both to personal safety (ability to satisfy daily needs with minimal physical and emotional risk) and medical safety (prevention of complications and access to medical services in case of emergency). The goal is to capitalize on patient, family, and community strengths; and to reach a consensus decision that effectively balances fulfillment of patient needs and patient and family values and preferences. Patient, family, and community contextual factors are very important considerations (see Table 6 in Chapter 3).

A therapeutic leave of absence (LOA) for the patient and a home visit by a therapist can greatly facilitate transition to an independent or assisted living situation in patients with moderate to severe residual disabilities. The LOA allows the patient and family to test their abilities and identify problem areas that require more attention before discharge. The home visit permits the therapist to identify safety hazards, rehearse the patient's daily routine, and assess the accessibility of community facilities typically used by the patient (e.g., a grocery store, church, or recreation center). When a home visit is not feasible, the strengths and limitations of the home environment need to be carefully reviewed during discussions with the patient and the family or other caregivers.

Minor structural problems at the chosen place of residence can be corrected by relocating storage of objects (e.g., clothing, grooming supplies, kitchen equipment and supplies, hobby equipment and supplies) or removing scatter rugs or obstacles to ambulation. Other problems may require purchase of equipment or alterations such as installation of a bath bench, toilet rails, or grab bars for the bath area, or widening doors to allow wheelchair access. Needs for major alterations (e.g., an elevator to enter the home or permit access to the second floor), strategies for improving access to community resources, and plans for action in case of emergency also can be reviewed.

Another important consideration in choosing a place of residence is making a realistic assessment of the caregiver support that will be available to the stroke survivor. This assessment can be aided by examining the contextual factors listed in Table 6 (see Chapter 3) and, where applicable, by repeating administration of the Family Assessment Device (see Attachment 12) to identify any interim changes that may affect the adequacy of support or indicate the need for family counseling. One cannot assume that a spouse, child, or friend with whom the patient was living before the stroke will be able or willing to provide needed support. For example, an elderly spouse who is in poor health may not be able to tolerate the physical and emotional strain of caregiving, and adult children may be unable or unwilling to take on caregiver responsibilities. If adequate support is not available at home, it may be necessary to look for an alternative place of residence. The role of caregiver and ways of assisting caregivers are discussed in the next chapter.

Patient and Family Education. Education and training of the patient and family prior to discharge should emphasize issues that will be most relevant during transition. These need to be individualized to the patient but may include:

- Preventing recurrent stroke.
- Signs and symptoms of potential complications.
- Signs and symptoms of psychological dysfunction.
- Medication taking.
- Techniques required for specific tasks (e.g., transfers, personal hygiene, and dressing).
- Swallowing techniques for the dysphagic patient.
- Nutrition and hydration.
- Care of an indwelling bladder catheter.
- Skin care.
- Use of a feeding tube.
- Home exercises.
- Sexual functioning.
- Recreational and vocational or volunteer pursuits.
- Driving a car.

Attention to family/caregiver education and counseling has been shown to increase knowledge, help stabilize some aspects of family functioning (Evans, Matlock, Bishop, et al., 1988), and contribute to the maintenance of rehabilitation gains (Garraway, Walton, Akhtar, et al., 1981; Strand, Asplund, Eriksson, et al., 1985).

Continuity of Care. All patients will require continued medical care after discharge from a rehabilitation program, and many patients will require continued rehabilitation services. Discharge planning includes making explicit arrangements for these services and ensuring that full information on the patient's medical and neurological status, the patient's responses to rehabilitation interventions, and recommendations for future medical and rehabilitation treatments are transmitted to future providers at the time of discharge. Effective communication will help avoid gaps in care and lay the groundwork for future progress. As discussed in the next chapter, a single health care provider should be in overall charge of coordinating medical and other services after discharge.

Community Services. Home care and other services from community agencies can help to supplement or substitute for services provided by family or caregivers. Some sources of community services are discussed in Chapter 7. Stroke groups, if available, may be particularly helpful to the patient and family. Every rehabilitation facility should maintain an up-to-date inventory of local, regional, and national services. These should be reviewed with the patient and family prior to discharge, and linkages should be established for services that are both needed and desired.

7 Transition to the Community

Living with disabilities after a stroke is a lifelong challenge during which people continue to seek and find ways to compensate for or adapt to persisting neurological deficits. For many stroke survivors and their families, the real work of recovery begins after formal rehabilitation. One of the most important tasks of a rehabilitation program is to help those involved to prepare for this stage of recovery.

Many people live on their own after a stroke. Others live with family members who will need to provide various kinds of support. The impact of every stroke is intensely individual, and each person and family has to chart a pathway to recovery. This chapter focuses mainly on the patient who lives with caregivers and on common themes that arise after return to a community residence.

The Transition Experience

The first few weeks after discharge from a rehabilitation program are often difficult, as the stroke survivor attempts to use newly learned skills without the support of the rehabilitation environment. Later on, other problems may emerge when the full impact of stroke becomes apparent as the person attempts to resume self-care activities and family relationships. Psychological and social effects of the stroke, such as communication disorders or limitations of short-term memory, are likely to become more obvious over time and may have profound effects on daily life.

Coping with this transition requires both preparedness and flexibility. The stroke survivor and family should be thoroughly prepared by discussion of transition issues before discharge, accompanied, whenever possible, by visits to the home by rehabilitation professionals to plan how specific activities will be accomplished. At the same time, they need to be able to respond to the unexpected. Most people rely on well-used, proven methods of problem solving that become automatic. During the first weeks following discharge from a program, stroke survivors and their caregivers may discover that familiar and comfortable approaches do not work well. This realization should be a cue to seek new information, insights, or resources. Flexibility and willingness to seek creative problem-solving methods will be the key.

Family and Caregiver Functioning

Recommendation: Clinicians need to be sensitive to potential adverse effects of caregiving on family functioning and the health of the caregiver. They should work with the patient and caregivers to avoid negative effects, promote problem solving, and facilitate reintegration

of the patient into valued family and social roles. (Research evidence=B; expert opinion=strong consensus.)

Support by family members or other caregivers is critical to achieving the best possible long-term outcomes for individuals with disabilities. The term **family** applies to people with whom the person has lived or will live, including extended family members. For older people, this will often be the spouse (but children, other relatives, or friends may also constitute the family). For younger people with stroke, parents and siblings may constitute the family unit. The term **caregiver** is used to identify the one or two individuals who provide most of the support, whether they are family members, close friends, or from a community agency. The majority of caregivers of stroke survivors are women.

Caring for a person with severe disabilities can be a formidable task. Impairments in mobility may tax an elderly spouse's physical strength and endurance; and cognitive, emotional, and communication problems often have pervasive effects on family and social relationships. In general, caregivers cope with physical limitations better than cognitive or emotional ones (Evans, 1986). However, even healthy and committed caregivers may "burn out" from the continuous pressure of providing support to a patient 24 hours a day, 7 days a week. Opportunities for respites may be extremely important.

Adverse health effects on caregivers have been well documented; they include increased risk of depression (Blazer, Hughes, and George, 1987; Kramer, German, Anthony, et al., 1985; Lichtenberg and Barth, 1990; Schultz, Uisintainer, and Williamson, 1990), increased use of health services, and the self-administration of medications prescribed originally for the stroke patient (Lichtenberg and Gibbons, 1992). Depression, in turn, has been associated with physical abuse of the patient (Joslin, Coyne, Johson, et al., 1991) and a greater likelihood of nursing home placement (Stephens, Kinney, and Igrocki, 1991). As many as 14 percent of employed caregivers of people with strokes have been reported to leave their jobs (Brocklehurst, Morris, Andrews, et al., 1981). Female caregivers are more likely to experience depression and serious lifestyle disruptions (Evans, Hendricks, Lawrence-Umlauf, et al., 1989).

Despite the difficulties, many caregivers and families function extremely well (Bishop, Epstein, Keitner, et al., 1986). Preexisting organizational and functional characteristics of the family may have important effects on the outcome (Bishop, Epstein, Keitner, et al., 1986; Evans, Bishop, Matlock, et al., 1987a and 1987b; Freidland and McColl, 1987; Gwyther and George, 1986; Jimenez and Morgan, 1979; Robinson, Bolduc, and Kubos, 1985; Susset, Vobecky, and Black, 1979). A caregiver is more likely to give adequate support if she or he is a spouse who is knowledgeable about stroke and its disabilities, is not depressed, and lives in an otherwise well-functioning family unit (Evans, Bishop, and Dusley, 1992). Families that have a history of adaptive coping, extensive social supports, and strong functional and affective mutuality usually function well. On the other hand, family patterns of constricted emotional responsiveness and rigid expectations about standards of behavior for cognitively impaired individuals are associated with more days of rehospitalization after a stroke (Evans, Bishop, Matlock, et al., 1987b). Pre-stroke family functioning has been shown to affect adherence to treatment (Evans, Bishop, Matlock, et al., 1987a), psychosocial adjustment (Evans, Bishop, Matlock, et al., 1987b), caregiver adjustment (Evans, Bishop, and Haselkorn, 1991), and the likelihood of nursing home placement (Evans and Noonan, 1988).

Cultural factors may have important effects on attitudes about disability, the roles of family members during transition, and the ability of the family to deal with the complexities of the health care system. Barriers may be especially difficult to circumvent if the family has a different cultural orientation from that of the community at large. Sensitive counseling can help families with decisions that run counter to traditional values.

Chapters 4 and 6 stressed the importance of patient and family/caregiver education during acute care and rehabilitation. Table 25 summarizes the results of studies of educational and support interventions offered during community transitions. The most impressive result was obtained by a study that examined the effects of reinforcing key educational messages and offering counseling to caregivers after the stroke survivor returns home (Evans, Matlock, Bishop, et al., 1988). In this study, one group of patients received education directed at improving the caregiver's ability to provide support, and another received education plus later counseling sessions to explore problems and reinforce previous education. Both experimental groups performed better than a control group, but benefits were sustained only in the group that received followup sessions. A related study demonstrated that participation of caregivers in *problem-solving* groups reduced the likelihood of depression compared to *supportive* groups (Lovett and Gallager, 1988).

Clinical followup should include assessment of caregiver and family functioning. An initial visit within 1 month of discharge will permit early identification of any problem areas and the development of education or counseling interventions to address them or efforts to obtain support from community sources. Responsibility for followup may rest with the stroke survivor's principal physician or may be delegated to a rehabilitation specialist who is providing continued services after discharge. Whoever performs this function, active involvement of the stroke survivor and family and continuity with previous education or counseling services are necessary.

Table 25. Evidence on the effectiveness of patient and family education and support interventions

Author Year Country	Purpose Study design Duration of deficits Number of subjects	Outcome measures Maximum followup	Conclusions/ comments
Friedland and McColl (1992) Canada	Determine if a social support intervention (SSI) increases support and psychosocial outcomes RCT Chronic deficits N=88	Social Support Inventory Interpersonal Support Evaluation List General Health Questionnaire (GHQ) Sickness Impact Profile (SIP) ADL (Barthel) F/U until 6 months	No significant differences among groups.
Jongbloed and Morgan (1991) Canada	Compare OT visits to assist in leisure activities to single OT home visit RCT Deficits < 15 months N=40	Katz Adjustment Index Free-time activities Satisfaction with activities F/U until 18 weeks	No significant differences.
Pain and McLellan (1990) United Kingdom	Test benefits of individualized booklets given to patients at discharge from rehabilitation RCT Duration of deficits not available N=36	ADL (Barthel) Frenchay Activities Index Caregiver Questionnaire F/U until 3 months	No significant differences on function or activities.
Towle, Lincoln, and Mayfield (1989) United Kingdom	Examine effects of a social worker intervention on use of health and social services RCT Chronic deficits N=44	Use of health and social services Financial benefits Extended ADL (EADL) Frenchay Activities Index F/U until 16 weeks	No significant differences on any measure.

See notes at end of table.

Table 25. Evidence on the effectiveness of patient and family education and support interventions (continued)

Author Year Country	Purpose Study design Duration of deficits Number of subjects	Outcome measures Maximum followup	Conclusions/ comments
Evans, Matlock, Bishop, et al. (1988) United States	Examine effects of caregiver education with and without additional counseling RCT Acute deficits N=188	Stroke Care Information Test (SCIT) Family Assessment Device (FAD) ESCROW Profile (social resources) Personal Adjustment and Role Skills Scale (PARS) F/U until 1 year	Both counseling and education significantly improved family functioning and caregiver knowledge. Counseling more effective than education alone and also resulted in better patient functioning. Neither intervention affected use of social resources.

Note: ADL = activities of daily living. F/U = followup. OT = occupational therapy. RCT = randomized controlled trial.

Continuity and Coordination of Patient Care

Recommendation: The stroke survivor's continuing care needs should be coordinated by a single physician or health care provider with the stroke survivor and the principal caregiver. (Research evidence=NA; expert opinion=strong consensus.)

The return to community living confronts the stroke survivor and caregivers with the sometimes formidable task of maintaining continuity with previous services and coordinating the broad range of medical, rehabilitative, and social services required by many persons with disabilities. Gaps in care will increase the risk of reinstitutionalization, and discontinuities in treatment regimens may slow progress toward functional independence. The importance of well-coordinated aftercare is accentuated by trends toward earlier discharges from both acute care and rehabilitation hospitals.

Responsibility for coordinating medical and health services during transition passes to the patient's principal physician or health care provider; outpatient or home care rehabilitation services often replace inpatient or nursing facility programs; and the stroke survivor and family/caregivers assume responsibility for daily activities. Each of these transitions requires careful planning and close communication among the parties involved.

The key players in the transition process are the stroke survivor, principal caregiver, and the primary physician or health care provider. The stroke survivor or the principal caregiver coordinates all issues, information, and actions. Occasionally, the physician, social worker, or visiting nurses will perform this function. This person should be identified as soon as possible after an acute stroke and should be fully knowledgeable concerning the stroke survivor's needs and resources.

The principal physician may be from any of a variety of medical specialties, but will most commonly be the patient's physician prior to the stroke or a rehabilitation specialist. This person is responsible for providing general medical services, coordinating medical specialty and rehabilitative services, and assessing the patient's progress. In many States, this person is legally required to certify disabilities and the patient's ability to drive an automobile. The advantages of involving a physician who is skilled in rehabilitation medicine should be considered, especially in the face of moderate or severe disabilities that require continued rehabilitation services.

Close communication among providers, the stroke survivor, and family/caregivers is essential at each stage. As a first step, a complete discharge summary should be given to the principal physician on the day of discharge. Table 26 lists the types of information that should be included.

Table 26. Information to be included in discharge summary following rehabilitation

- Patient's medical history, including functional status prior to stroke and on admission to rehabilitation.
- Current physical examination and clinical course including complications experienced, diagnoses, and current medical and rehabilitative treatment regimens.
- Type, intensity, and duration of interventions received during rehabilitation and functional responses to these.
- Continuing requirements for support in mobility, functional health patterns, and performance of self-care activities.
- Anticipated need for medical care and equipment.
- Cognitive, psychological, or behavioral problems experienced, their current treatments, and anticipated future problems.
- Specific recommendations for continued rehabilitation services and a "best estimate" of the functional prognosis.

Subsequently, all clinical information should be centralized in a single patient record. This should include information on progress during rehabilitation therapies and progress toward functional independence, as well as on medical and other health conditions.

Recommendation: An initial visit with the stroke survivor's principal physician or health care providers should be scheduled within 1 month of discharge from an inpatient rehabilitation program or sooner if necessary. (Research evidence=NA; expert opinion=strong consensus.)

To promote continuity of care, appointments with the principal physician and with needed outpatient or home rehabilitation services should be arranged at the time of discharge. An initial followup visit should be scheduled within 1 month of discharge unless medical conditions require earlier attention. In addition, the stroke survivor and family/caregiver should be given a phone contact (hotline) to a person who is familiar with the stroke survivor's condition and should be encouraged to use this at any time if questions or problems arise. Depending on the circumstances, this phone contact may be with the principal physician's office, the discharging rehabilitation program, the visiting nurse, or the community agency providing the services.

Postdischarge Monitoring

Recommendation: The stroke survivor's progress should be evaluated within 1 month after return to a community residence and at regular intervals during at least the first year, consistent with the person's condition and the preferences of the stroke survivor and family. Monitoring of physical, cognitive, and emotional functioning and integration into family and social roles is especially important. (Research evidence=NA; expert opinion=strong consensus.)

The goals of monitoring are to document whether the stroke survivor is maintaining the functional gains achieved during rehabilitation, making further progress toward functional independence, and reintegrating successfully with the family and community. The period following return to the community is a high-risk time. Gaps in care may occur as responsibility shifts from the rehabilitation program to the principal physician, other rehabilitation services, or community agencies. Moreover, emotional stress, exacerbation of medical conditions, and difficulty in sustaining the level of activities achieved during rehabilitation are common. Regression may occur because of lack of stimulation, lack of confidence, or a physical environment that makes daily activities difficult to perform, or if the family/caregivers inadvertently suppress initiative by *taking over* rather than *encouraging* self-performance of activities.

The purpose of postdischarge assessment is to obtain the information needed to guide medical care, promote adjustment to the living environment, identify needs for additional rehabilitation services, and improve the ability of the family or other caregivers to provide support. Types of information to be obtained are identified in Table 27. Especially important are measures of success in adapting to the living environment and functioning independently, adherence to medical and rehabilitation regimens, and the ability of caregivers to provide needed support.

Table 27. Assessment after return to the community

General clinical assessment: neurological and medical examinations
■ Neurological deficits. ■ Comorbid diseases. ■ Stroke-related risk factors. ■ Affective disorders. ■ Adherence to medical and rehabilitation regimens. ■ Functional health patterns: nutrition and hydration, ability to swallow, bowel and bladder continence, skin integrity, activity tolerance, sleep patterns.
Adaptation to environment
■ Patient adaptation and functional performance. ■ Family/caregiver functioning.
Standardized instruments (numbers in parentheses refer to attachment tables in this guideline)
■ Measure of disability (ADL) (4). ■ Instrumental activities of daily living (IADL) scale (11). ■ Family Assessment Device (12). ■ Quality-of-life scale (13).

Note: ADL = activities of daily living.

The use of standardized tests is recommended to evaluate ADL and IADL performance, quality of life, and family functioning. Identification of problem areas in personal or family functioning may indicate the need for additional psychological or social support. A quality-of-life scale is included to assess general well-being and life satisfaction and to identify priorities for future treatment. These instruments should be used in a consistent fashion from one examination to the next, and should be administered by people who are well trained in their administration.

Responsibility for monitoring progress rests with the principal physician, though responsibility for collecting clinical data may be shared with rehabilitation clinicians or community agencies. Evaluations can be performed at the time of medical or rehabilitation visits and can be supplemented by telephone interviews with the stroke survivor or a family member. Initially, a home visit is preferable for patients who remain moderately or severely disabled because of the valuable insights that direct observation can provide into how the individual and family members actually function. The initial evaluation should be performed at the time of the first scheduled followup visit with the physician, within 1 month of discharge. Thereafter, the frequency of evaluation will depend on the needs of the stroke survivor and the family/caregivers. Objectives are to identify areas of disability that may benefit from additional medical or rehabilitation services, counseling, or community services, and to obtain the objective evidence of progress needed to justify continuation of rehabilitation services.

Continued Rehabilitation Services

Recommendation: Continued rehabilitation services should be considered to help the stroke survivor sustain the gains from the rehabilitation program and to build on patient and family strengths and interests as that patient becomes reintegrated into the home and community. Services should be phased out as measurable benefit diminishes. (Research evidence=NA; expert opinion=consensus.)

Continued rehabilitation services can provide a bridge between the protected environment of the rehabilitation program and independent living. Decisions about such services will depend on the patient's progress during the preceding rehabilitation program and on the level of remaining disabilities. A gradual withdrawal of services rather than sudden cessation is often preferable, since an abrupt end to professional services is often interpreted by patients as an end to improvement (Doolittle, 1992). Followup visits help to identify problems encountered during transition, reinforce expectations of long-term progress, and permit development of a plan to achieve functional independence after the withdrawal of services.

Continued rehabilitation should take full advantage of the patient's and family's strengths and interests, and interventions should be directed at areas of function and activities that are particularly high priorities. These might include, for example, valued hobbies or recreational activities, social relationships, and preexisting family roles. A strong ethnic orientation might provide access to community activities or social groups. The contextual issues summarized in Table 6 (see Chapter 3) become particularly important during transition.

Community Supports

Recommendation: Acute care hospitals and rehabilitation facilities should maintain up-to-date inventories of community resources, provide this information to stroke survivors and their families/caregivers, and offer assistance in obtaining needed services. (Research evidence=NA; expert opinion=strong consensus.)

Community supports can help buffer the effects of disabilities on the patient and family/caregivers. Broadly, supports can be categorized as educational, instrumental, or emotional. Educational supports include printed materials, videotapes, computer programs, and information on support groups available from individuals or health professionals, or through organizations such as the American Heart Association and National Stroke Association. Instrumental support refers to physical services such as homemaker services and Meals on Wheels or devices such as ramps or wheelchairs. Emotional support is a broad concept that intrinsically involves people: people to talk to, to turn to for advice, or to seek counsel from. Having people to turn to has been shown to be beneficial even when the advice is rejected (McFarlane, Norman, Streiner, et al., 1983). Strong social support has been shown to improve outcomes, especially in patients with severe strokes (Glass, Matchar, Belyea, et al., 1993). Great attention should be given to opportunities and methods for improving the effectiveness of social support. One such direction is to facilitate linkages and transfer of information between self-help groups and the health care system (Borkman, 1990).

Most social support comes from family, caregivers, and friends. The tendency, however, is for friends and relatives to rally around after the acute stroke, but then dissipate, leaving the person and immediate family to become increasingly isolated over the longer term. Community resources become especially important under these circumstances. Table 28 identifies some national and regional organizations that provide support to persons with stroke and their families. Most of these have local offices or branches in many communities. Availability of additional local resources will vary from community to community. Acute care hospitals and rehabilitation facilities will provide a valuable service if they maintain up-to-date inventories of available resources, and help stroke survivors and families gain access to them.

Safety and Health Promotion During Transition

Fall Prevention

Recommendation: Fall prevention after the stroke survivor returns to a community residence should emphasize identifying patient, treatment, and environmental risk factors, and steps to reduce these risks. (Research evidence=C; expert opinion=strong consensus.)

The efforts of stroke survivors to increase mobility inevitably increase the risk of falls. The goal is to minimize these risks while encouraging efforts to achieve independence. Potentially remediable risk factors include residual muscle weakness, problems with balance or gait, problems with vision, orthostatic hypotension, overuse of sedatives, medication side effects, and inappropriate assistive devices or inadequate training in their use (Rubenstein, Robbins, Josephson, et al., 1990). Environmental hazards such as scatter rugs, elevated thresholds, unsafe placement of furniture, and inadequate lighting are also important.

Table 28. Resources for stroke survivors and families/caregivers

ACTION 1100 Vermont Avenue NW Washington, DC 20525 Telephone: (202) 606-4855 Call for number of regional office	A Federal Agency. Sponsors older American volunteer programs. These include: ■ Retired Senior Volunteer Program (RSVP). People age 55 and over are volunteers in schools, libraries, hospitals, and other community settings. ■ Senior Companion Program. Volunteers (any age) provide assistance so that low-income people age 60 and over can remain in their homes. ■ Foster Grandparent Program. Low-income people age 60 and over are volunteers caring for children with special needs.
Administration on Aging 330 Independence Avenue SW Washington, DC 20201 Telephone: toll-free (800) 677-1116 (Eldercare Locator Number) Call for list of community services for elders in local area	An Agency of the Department of Health and Human Services. Provides community services for people age 60 and over (and spouses, regardless of age). Services are provided by State and area agencies on aging. Services helpful to stroke survivors and families include homemaker services, Meals on Wheels (meals delivered to the home), congregate dining (group meals in a senior center or other community setting), transportation, senior center activities, and information and referrals.
AHA Stroke Connection (formerly the Courage Stroke Network) American Heart Association 7272 Greenville Avenue Dallas, TX 75231-4596 Telephone: toll-free (800) 553-6321 Or, check telephone book for local AHA office	Operates through national office and through local American Heart Association offices. Provides: ■ Educational books, pamphlets, videos, and tapes about stroke for stroke survivors and for families and caregivers. ■ Referral to stroke clubs or other self-help groups in stroke survivor's local area. ■ Help in starting stroke clubs and other self-help groups. ■ *Stroke Connection* newsletter for stroke survivors and caregivers. ■ *Stroke of Luck* newsletter for stroke survivors with aphasia and caregivers.

Table 28. Resources for stroke survivors and families/caregivers (continued)

American Dietetic Association/National Center for Nutrition and Dietetics 216 West Jackson Boulevard Chicago, IL 60606-6995 Telephone: toll-free (800) 366-1655 (Consumer Nutrition Hotline)	Promotes optimal nutrition, health, and well-being for consumers through its various programs and services: ■ Consumers may speak to a registered dietitian for answers to nutrition questions, or obtain a referral to a local registered dietitian.
American Self-Help Clearinghouse St. Clares-Riverside Medical Center Denville, NJ 07834 Telephone: (201) 625-7101 Call for name and number of State or local clearinghouse	Operates through State and local clearinghouses. Provides information on local self-help groups and assistance in starting a self-help group.
National Aphasia Association P.O. Box 1887 Murray Hill Station New York, NY 10156-0611 Telephone: toll-free (800) 922-4622	Operates through national office and local affiliates and promotes national awareness. Provides: ■ Educational books and pamphlets about aphasia. ■ Referral to community services.
National Easter Seal Society 230 West Monroe Street, Suite 1800 Chicago, IL 60606 Telephone: (312) 726-6200 Or, check telephone book for local Easter Seal Society	Provides information and services to help people with disabilities, including those from stroke. Operates through national office and local Easter Seal Societies. Provides: ■ Educational books, pamphlets, and audiovisual aids about disabilities. ■ Posters and other publicity to educate the public about people with disabilities. ■ Rehabilitation services including physical, occupational, and speech therapy. ■ Guidance about assistive devices (such as wheelchairs). ■ Vocational evaluation, training, and placement. ■ Recreational and social services. ■ Catalog of publications and products.

Table 28. Resources for stroke survivors and families/caregivers (continued)

National Stroke Association 8480 East Orchard Road, Suite 1000 Englewood, CO 80111-5015 Telephone: (303) 771-1700 Toll-free (800) STROKES (787-6537)	Promotes stroke prevention, treatment, rehabilitation, family support, and research. Provides: ■ Educational books, pamphlets, and audiovisual materials about stroke for stroke survivors, families, and caregivers. ■ Information on local stroke clubs and other self-help groups. ■ Support for stroke research. ■ Training programs about stroke for health care professionals. ■ *Be Stroke Smart* newsletter for stroke survivors, families/caregivers, and health care professionals.
Rosalynn Carter Institute Georgia Southwestern College 600 Simmons Street Americus, GA 31709	Provides information on caregiving. Reading lists, video products, and other caregiver resources are available by writing to the address listed at left.
Stroke Clubs International 805 12th Street Galveston, TX 77550 Telephone: (409) 762-1022	Run by stroke survivors. Promotes hiring of people with disabilities. Provides lists of stroke clubs in each State.
The Well Spouse Foundation P.O. Box 801 New York, NY 10023 Telephone: (212) 724-7209 Toll-free (800) 838-0879	Provides support for the husbands, wives, and partners of people who are chronically ill or disabled. Provides bimonthly newsletter, regional support groups, pen pal system, and an advocacy program.

Fall prevention may include exercise regimens that increase muscle strength and improve postural control, modification of medication regimens, careful attention to the selection and use of assistive devices and wheelchairs, and home modifications to reduce the risk of tripping and increase the ease with which a person can perform daily activities. Improved access to bathroom facilities will be particularly helpful in reducing the risk of falls. A well-designed fall prevention program has been shown to reduce falls by 9 percent, rehospitalization by 26 percent, and hospital days by 52 percent (Rubenstein, Robbins, Josephson, et al., 1990).

Injuries from falls and the fear of falling may both impede recovery. Fall prevention needs to aim at both physical and psychological outcomes. Teaching the stroke survivor and family members techniques for getting up after a fall can help reduce anxiety.

Health Promotion

Recommendation: High priority should be given to the prevention of stroke recurrence and stroke complications and to health promotion more generally, after the stroke survivor returns to the community. (Research evidence=A; expert opinion=strong consensus.)

The risk of suffering a second stroke averages 7 to 10 percent per year, and the risk of complications remains high, especially in severely disabled people with limited mobility. Interventions to prevent stroke recurrence and complications of stroke such as urinary tract infections, aspiration, pressure ulcers, DVT, and pulmonary emboli were discussed in Chapter 4. Continued efforts to prevent recurrent strokes are essential. The choice of therapies will depend on the etiology of the stroke and the stroke survivor's risk-factor profile. Steps to control risk factors such as hypertension, tobacco use, diabetes mellitus, hyperlipidemia, and drug abuse should be pursued. Timely vaccinations to prevent influenza and pneumococcal infection are very important in older patients.

Resuming Valued Activities

Leisure and Recreational Activities

Recommendation: Valued leisure activities should be identified, encouraged, and enabled. (Research evidence=C; expert opinion=strong consensus.)

Participation in leisure activities is closely related to both health status and quality of life (Drummond, 1990; Jongbloed and Morgan, 1991; Krefting and Krefting, 1991; Shank, 1992; Sjogren, 1982). Emphasis on leisure activities during rehabilitation can reinforce treatments directed at physical, emotional, and cognitive impairments or disabilities (MacNeil and Pringnitz, 1982). After return home, interest in leisure and recreational activities may provide a strong motivation to resume an active lifestyle. The support of family members and friends should be mobilized to influence a person's self-appraisal, roles, and participation in leisure activities.

Several measures of leisure activities have been developed (Holbrook and Skilbeck, 1983; Wade, Legh-Smith, and Langton-Hewer, 1985). Broadly, efforts to assess, encourage, and enable leisure and recreational activities after the stroke survivor returns home should include:

- Assessment of pre-stroke interests and activities.
- Agreement on short-term and longer-term goals.
- Review of valued activities against current functional levels.
- Evaluation of the suitability of current adaptive equipment.
- Development of strategies to overcome physical barriers in the home and community.

- Identification of new leisure activities to match functional abilities.
- Education concerning available community resources.
- When needed, advocacy for the development of community programs.

In addition to purely recreational activities, stroke survivors may be interested in opportunities for volunteer work. Volunteer activities not only can be rewarding in themselves, but also can provide a transition to paid employment for some people.

Sexuality

Recommendation: Sexual issues should be discussed during rehabilitation and addressed again after transition to the community when the stroke survivor and significant other are ready. (Research evidence=NA; Expert opinion=strong consensus.)

Sexual issues relate both to sexual function and to changes in body image as a result of stroke. Sexual activity usually diminishes and sometimes ceases after stroke (Bray, DeFrank, and Wolfe, 1981; Coslett and Heilman, 1986; Kalliomaki, Markkanen, and Mustonen, 1961), but sex remains important to the majority of stroke survivors. Decreases in libido or the ability to achieve orgasm are common after stroke (Coslett and Heilman, 1986; Garlinghouse, 1987). Men may experience difficulty in achieving an erection or ejaculating due to neurological impairments or the effects of medications, most notably those used to treat hypertension and cardiac disease; and women may experience changes that cause them to feel equally impotent. Psychological factors, dependency in self-care activities, and changes in sexual roles each may be important.

Sexual issues are often not adequately addressed despite evidence that patients and their partners welcome frank discussions. The most important message is that sexual activity is not contraindicated after stroke. However, both parties need to recognize and adjust for the effects of motor, sensory, and attentional deficits, easy fatigability, changes in body image, and self-esteem. Interventions that stress the importance of effective communication, sharing of concerns, and development of adaptive strategies such as positioning, foreplay, and timing to avoid fatigue are often helpful (McCormick, Riffer, and Thompson, 1986; Sjogren, Damber, and Liliequist, 1983; Sjogren and Fugl-Meyer, 1982).

Automobile Driving

Recommendation: Assessment of the ability of a disabled stroke survivor to drive a car should be based on a neurological examination, behavioral observations, and evaluation by the State agency responsible for issuing drivers' licenses (including a standardized driving test). Neuropsychological testing should be obtained in persons with cognitive or behavioral disorders. Referral to adaptive driving

instruction should be considered. (Research evidence=C; expert opinion=consensus.)

More than half of stroke survivors who drove a car before their strokes stop driving afterwards (Legh-Smith, Wade, and Hewer, 1986). Factors that are most commonly associated with driving cessation are older age and the presence of cognitive deficits. The ability to resume driving promotes independence and can also help greatly to avoid a sense of isolation.

Studies have come to mixed conclusions about the relative merits of neuropsychological examinations and standardized driving tests in evaluating persons with disabilities who wish to resume driving. Some studies suggest that persons who pass tests for cognitive deficits (including visuospatial deficits) do not require a road test (Nouri, Tinson, and Lincoln, 1987; Sivak, Olsen, Kewman, et al., 1981). Other studies find that cognitive testing alone is insufficient and recommend that a standardized driving test be mandatory (Brooke, Questad, Patterson, et al., 1992; Katz, Golden, Butter, et al., 1990; van Zomeren, Brouwer, and Minderhoud, 1987).

The panel's recommendations reflect the fact that stroke survivors may be able to pass a driving test despite having visuospatial deficits or problems with easy distractibility, impulsive behaviors, or slowed decisionmaking that may impair their ability to drive safely under unpredictable road conditions. These problems will usually be detected during rehabilitation. If questions persist, however, a neuropsychological evaluation should be obtained prior to the driving test.

Decisions on a stroke survivor's ability to drive also need to take account of medical problems such as the control of seizures, and must satisfy local regulations that govern driving with an impairment or medical condition. Referral to an adaptive driving instruction program should be considered in appropriate patients. The only study that has examined the effectiveness of cognitive potential training concluded that training may improve perceptual skills and driving performance (Sivak, Hill, Henson, et al., 1984).

The final authority on whether a person is allowed to drive is the bureau or department of motor vehicles or other agency responsible in each State for issuing driver's licenses. The person who has had a stroke and wishes to resume driving should inform that agency and seek validation of his or her ability to drive safely. The person's insurance company should also be notified both about the stroke and about the subsequent validation of driving ability from the State agency.

Returning to Work

Recommendation: Stroke survivors who worked prior to their strokes should, if their condition permits, be encouraged to be evaluated for

the potential to return to work. Vocational counseling should be offered when appropriate. (Research evidence=NA; expert opinion=consensus.)

The ability of a person to pursue a vocation is an important determinant of the quality of life. This is as true for older people who would like to work as it is for younger people. The 1986 ICD Survey of Disabled Americans, in fact, stated that "not working is perhaps the truest definition of what it means to be disabled" (Louis Harris and Associates, 1986). The Americans with Disabilities Act of 1990 prohibits discrimination in employment against people with disabilities.

Vocational rehabilitation has been congressionally mandated for over 50 years to provide permanently disabled people with whatever assistance is necessary to prepare them for work that they can do successfully. However, a population survey published by the U.S. Census Bureau in 1988 revealed that only 32 percent of working-age adults with disabilities were working or actively seeking employment.

Barriers to Vocational Reintegration. There are many barriers to successful vocational reintegration of individuals with disabilities from stroke. These include:

- Lack of knowledge about stroke and its consequences among stroke survivors, their families, communities, potential employers, and community-based social service and allied health professionals.
- Architectural barriers in the workplace.
- Limited access to appropriate vocational rehabilitation resources in communities distant from major rehabilitation facilities.
- Limited awareness of vocational services on the part of health professionals (Smolkin and Cohen, 1974).
- Negative attitudes of some health professionals toward return to work by stroke survivors (Smolkin and Cohen, 1974).
- Misunderstanding and negative attitudes on the part of stroke survivors and families toward vocational rehabilitation as a result of lack of information on the services available and how to obtain them.
- Depression or other emotional problems affecting the motivation and ability of a stroke survivor to seek employment.
- Financial disincentives in such areas as health insurance coverage, disability payments, and costs of environmental adaptions and transportation.
- Inefficiency or lack of interest of vocational rehabilitation programs in dealing with stroke survivors.

Major Needs for Vocational Rehabilitation. To serve stroke survivors effectively, the vocational rehabilitation system needs to improve assessment, interventions, patient education, and patient advocacy.

Traditional vocational assessment methodologies may close off opportunities for stroke survivors with behavioral or cognitive deficits and result in low-paying, unsatisfying jobs (Nadolsky, 1985). Flexible assessment and placement models are needed that take account of a variety of personal, medical, psychological, educational, work history, community, and economic variables—and are firmly rooted in real work and living situations. None of the evaluation tools available to help determine a person's readiness for vocational rehabilitation have been validated in patients with stroke. The better known tools include: a Vocational Assessment Protocol (VAP) (Thomas, 1990), Work Performance Assessment (WPA), McCarron-Dial Perceptual Memory Task (PMJ) (Chan, Lynch, Dial, et al., 1993), Work and the Supervisors Rating Scale and Functional Assessment Inventory (Crowe and Athelestan, 1981).

Vocational interventions traditionally follow the medical model that sequentially evaluates deficits, prescribes treatments to fix the problems, tests the solution within a prescribed range of job options, and recycles the client if the initial placement fails. Client-centered services would depart from this approach by eliciting the full partnership of the stroke survivor and family/caregiver from the beginning, and by retaining flexibility to change objectives and strategies as the person's capabilities grow or the work environment changes. The ability of the program to build skills and to offer retraining programs may be particularly important in helping the stroke survivor find employment.

The greatest opportunities for clinicians to support vocational reintegration are in the areas of education and advocacy. Clinicians should be prepared to assist persons who have been disabled by strokes and wish to examine the possibility of returning to work. They should make sure that these people are given complete information on available vocational rehabilitation programs, are helped in gaining access to these, and receive an assessment of their potential to return to work that takes into account prior employment, present physical condition, psychological and social status, and motivation.

In addition, both clinicians and vocational rehabilitation professionals should talk with employers to encourage them to hire people with disabilities from stroke or other causes. Myths about negative effects of disabilities on work productivity need to be dispelled. Vocational rehabilitation professionals should provide technical assistance to employers in conducting job analyses, writing job descriptions, and providing job accommodations that are appropriate to employees who have had strokes.

References

Adams HP, Bendixen BH, Kappelle J, Biller J, Love BB, Gordon DL, Marsh EE, and the TOAST Investigators. Classification of subtype of acute ischemic stroke. Stroke 1993;24:35–41.

Adams HP, Brott TG, Crowell RM, Furlan AJ, et al., editors. Management of patients with acute ischemic stroke. Dallas (TX): American Heart Association; 1994.

Ahlsio B, Britton M, Murray V, Theorell T. Disablement and quality of life after stroke. Stroke 1984 Sep-Oct;15(5):886–90.

American Heart Association. Heart and stroke facts. Dallas (TX): American Heart Association; 1991.

Andersen G, Verstergaard K, Lauritzen L. Effective treatment of poststroke depression with the selective serotonin reuptake inhibitor citalopram. Stroke 1994;25:1099–109.

Anderson S, Tranel D. Awareness of disease states following cerebral infarction, dementia and head trauma: standardized assessment. Clin Neuropsychologist 1989;3:327–39.

Andrews K, Brocklehurst JC, Richards B, Laycock PJ. The rate of recovery from stroke—and its measurement. Int Rehabil Med 1981;3(3):155–61.

Asberg KH. Orthostatic tolerance training of stroke patients in general medical wards. An experimental study. Scand J Rehabil Med 1989;21(4):179–85.

Awad EA, Dykstra D. Treatment of spasticity by neurolysis. In: Kottke FJ, Lehmann JF, editors. Krusen's handbook of physical medicine and rehabilitation. 4th ed. Philadelphia: WB Saunders; 1990. p. 1154–61.

Axelsson K, Asplund K, Norberg A, Alafuzoff I. Nutritional status in patients with acute stroke. Acta Med Scand 1988;224(3):217–24.

Axelsson K, Asplund K, Norberg A, Alafuzoff I. Nutritional status in patients with acute stroke. The implications of cognitive adaptation and social support ideas for coping with a stroke are discussed. Soc Sci Med 1989;28(3):239–47.

Bachman DL, Wolf PA, Linn RT, Knoefel JE, Cobb JL, Belanger AJ, White LR, D'Agostino RB. Incidence of dementia and probable Alzheimer's disease in a general population: the Framingham Study. Neurology 1993;43:515–9.

Bamford J, Sandercock P, Dennis M, Warlow C. A prospective study of acute cerebrovascular disease in the community: the Oxfordshire Community Stroke Project: 2. Incidence, case fatality rates and overall outcome at one year of cerebral infarction, primary intracerebral and subarachnoid hemorrhage. J Neurology and Psychiatry 1990;53:16–22.

Basmajian JV, Gowland C, Brandstater ME, Swanson L, Trotter J. EMG feedback treatment of upper limb in hemiplegic stroke patients: a pilot study. Arch Phys Med Rehabil 1982 Dec;63(12):613–6.

Basmajian JV, Gowland CA, Finlayson MA, Hall AL, Swanson LR, Stratford PW, Trotter JE, Brandstater ME. Stroke treatment: comparison of integrated behavioral-physical therapy vs traditional physical therapy programs. Arch Phys Med Rehabil 1987 May;68(5 Pt 1):267–72.

Basmajian JV, Kukulka CG, Narayan MG, Takebe K. Biofeedback treatment of foot-drop after stroke compared with standard rehabilitation technique: effects on voluntary control and strength. Arch Phys Med Rehabil 1975 Jun;56(6):231–6.

Basso A, Capitani E, Vignolo LA. Influence of rehabilitation on language skills in aphasic patients. A controlled study. Arch Neurol 1979 Apr;36(4):190–6.

Beck AT, Steer RA. Beck Depression Inventory: manual. Rev. ed., New York: NY Psychological Corporation; 1987.

Beck AT, Ward CH, Mendelson M, Mock J, Erbaugh J. An inventory for measuring depression. Arch Gen Psychiatry 1961 Jun;4:561–71.

Bellavance A, for the Ticlopidine Aspirin Stroke Study Group. Efficacy of ticlopidine and aspirin for prevention of reversible cerebrovascular ischemic events. The Ticlopidine Aspirin Stroke Study. Stroke 1993;24:1452–7.

Bennett CJ, Diokno AC. Clean intermittent self catheterization in the elderly. Urology 1984;24(1):43–5.

Ben-Yishay Y, Diller L, Gerstman L, Haas A. The relationship between impersistence, intellectual function and outcome of rehabilitation in patients with left hemiplegia. Neurology 1968 Sep;18(9):852–61.

Ben-Yishay Y, Gerstman L, Diller L, Haas A. Prediction of rehabilitation outcomes from psychometric parameters in left hemiplegics. J Consult Clin Psychol 1970 Jun;34(3):436–41.

Berg K. Measuring balance in the elderly: development and validation of an instrument. MSc thesis, McGill University; 1988.

Berg K. Measuring balance in the elderly: validation of an instrument. PhD thesis, McGill University; 1993.

Berg K, Maki B, Williams JI, Holliday P, Wood-Dauphinee S. A comparison of clinical and laboratory measures of postural balance in an elderly population. Arch Phys Med Rehabil 1992;73:1073–83.

Berg K, Wood-Dauphinee S, Williams JI, Gayton D. Measuring balance in the elderly: preliminary development of an instrument. Physiother Can 1989;41:304–11.

Berg K, Wood-Dauphinee S, Williams JI, Maki B. Measuring balance in the elderly: validation of an instrument. Can J Public Health 1992 Jul-Aug Suppl 2:S7–11.

Berglund K, Fugl-Meyer AR. Upper extremity function in hemiplegia. A cross-validation study of two assessment methods. Scand J Rehabil Med 1986;18(4):155–7.

Bergner M, Bobbitt RA, Carter WB, Gilson BS. The Sickness Impact Profile: development and final revision of a health status measure. Med Care 1981;19:787–805.

Bergstrom G, Aniansson A, Bjelle A, Grimby G, Lundgre B, Svanborg A. Functional consequences of joint impairment at age 79. Scand J Rehab Med 1985;17:183–90.

Bergstrom N, Braden BJ, Laguzza A, Holman V. The Braden Scale for predicting pressure sore risk. Nurs Res 1987 Jul-Aug;36(4):205–10.

Bergstrom N, Demuth PJ, Braden BJ. A clinical trial of the Braden Scale for predicting pressure sore risk. Nurs Clin North Am 1987 Jun;22(2):417–28.

Beyerman K. In: Mclane AM, editor. Conference on the classification of nursing diagnosis. 7th ed. St Louis (MO): CV Mosby; 1987.

Bishop DS, Epstein NB, Keitner GI, Miller IW, Srinivasan SV. Stroke: morale, family functioning, health status, and functional capacity. Arch Phys Med Rehabil 1986 Feb;67(2):84–7.

Bjork DT, Pelletier LL, Tight RR. Urinary tract infections with antibiotic resistant organisms in catheterized nursing home patients. Infect Control 1984;5(4):173–6.

Blazer D, Hughes D, George L. The epidemiology of depression in an elderly community population. Gerontologist 1987;27:281–7.

Bobath B. Adult hemiplegia: evaluation and treatment. 3rd ed. London: William Hinneman Medical Books; 1990.

Bobath B. Hemiplegia: evaluation and treatment. 2nd ed. Oxford; Boston: Butterworth-Heinemann; 1978.

Bolla-Wilson K, Robinson RG, Starkstein SE, Boston J, Price TR. Lateralization of dementia of depression in stroke patients. Am J Psychiatry 1989 May;146(5):627–34.

Bonita R, Beaglehole R. Recovery of motor function after stroke. Stroke 1988 Dec;19(12):1497–500.

Bonita R, Beaglehole R, North JDK. Event, incidence and case fatality rates of cerebrovascular disease in Auckland, New Zealand. Am J Epidemiol 1984;120:236–43.

Bonita R, Steward A, Beaglehole R. International trends in stroke mortality: 1970-1985. Stroke 1990;21:989–92.

Borgman MF, Passarella PM. Nursing care of the stroke patient using Bobath principles. An approach to altered movement. Nurs Clin North Am 1991 Dec;26(4):1019–35.

Borkman T. Self-help groups at the turning point: emerging egalitarian alliances with the formal health care system? Am J Community Psychol 1990;18(2):321–32.

Boston area anticoagulation trial for atrial fibrillation. The effect of low-dose warfarin on the risk of stroke in patients with non-rheumatic atrial fibrillation. N Engl J Med 1990;323:1504–11.

Bounds JV, Wiebers DO, Whisnant JP, Okazaki H. Mechanisms and timing of deaths from cerebral infarction. Stroke 1981;12:474–7.

Bowman BR, Baker LL, Waters RL. Positional feedback and electrical stimulation: an automated treatment for the hemiplegic wrist. Arch Phys Med Rehabil 1979 Nov;60(11):497–502.

Braden BJ. Clinical utility of the Braden Scale for predicting pressure sore risk. Decubitus 1989 Aug;2(3):44–6, 50–1.

Braden B, Bergstrom N. Braden Scale for predicting pressure ulcers in adults. Pressure ulcers in adults: prediction and prevention. Clinical practice guideline, no. 3. AHCPR publication no. 92-0047. Rockville (MD): Agency for Health Care Policy and Research. May 1992. p. 16–7.

Braden B, Bergstrom N. A conceptual schema for the study of the etiology of pressure sores. Rehabil Nurs 1987 Jan-Feb;12(1):8–12.

Branch LG, Jette AM. The Framingham Disability Study. I. Social disability among the aging. Am J Public Health 1981;71:1202–10.

Brandstater M, Basmajian J. Stroke rehabilitation. Baltimore (MD): Williams & Wilkins; 1987.

Brandstater ME, de Bruin H, Gowland C, Clark BM. Hemiplegic gait: analysis of temporal variables. Arch Phys Med Rehabil 1983 Dec;64(12):583–7.

Brandstater ME, Roth EJ, Siebens HC. Venous thromboembolism in stroke: literature review and implications for clinical practice. Arch Phys Med Rehabil 1992;73 (Suppl):379–89.

Bray GP, DeFrank RS, Wolfe TL. Sexual functioning in stroke survivors. Arch Phys Med Rehabil 1981 Jun;62(6):286–8.

Brocklehurst JC, Andrews K, Richards B, Laycock PJ. Incidence and correlates of incontinence in stroke patients. J Am Geriatr Soc 1985 Aug;33(8):540–2.

Brocklehurst JC, Morris P, Andrews K, Richards B, Laycock P. Social effects of stroke. Soc Sci Med 1981 Jan;15(A):35–9.

Broderick JP, Phillips SJ, Whisnant JP, O'Fallon WM, Bergstralh EJ. Incidence rates of stroke in the eighties: the end of the decline in stroke. Stroke 1989;20:577–82.

Brooke MM, Questad KA, Patterson DR, Valois TA. Driving evaluation after traumatic brain injury. Am J Phys Med Rehabil 1992;71:177–82.

Brott T, Adams HP, Olinger CP, Marler JR, Barsan WG, Biller J, Spilker J, Holleran R, Eberle R, Hertzberg V, et al. Measurements of acute cerebral infarction: a clinical examination scale. Stroke 1989 Jul;20(7):864–70.

Burnside IG, Tobias HS, Bursill D. Electromyographic feedback in the remobilization of stroke patients: a controlled trial. Arch Phys Med Rehabil 1982 May;63(5):217–22.

Butfield E, Zangwill O. Re-education in aphasia: a review of 70 cases. J Neurol Neurosurg Psychiatry 1946:75–9.

Butland RJA, Pang J, Gross ER, Woodcock AA, Geddes DM. Two, six and twelve minute walking tests in respiratory disease. BMJ 1982;284:1604–8.

Butter CE, Kirsh N. Combined and separate effects of eye patching and visual stimulation on unilateral neglect following stroke. Arch Phys Med Rehabil 1992;73:1133–9.

Butter CM, Kirsch NL, Reeves G. The effect of lateralised stimuli on unilateral spatial neglect following right hemisphere lesions. Restorative Neurology and Neuroscience 1990;2:39–46.

Byles J, Bryne C, Boyle M, Offord D. Ontario child health study: reliability and validity of the general functioning subscale of the McMaster Family Assessment Device. Family Process 1988;27:97–104.

Byng S. Sentence processing deficits: theory and therapy. Cognitive Neuropsychology 1988;5:629–76.

Carey JR. Manual stretch: effect on finger movement control and force control in stroke subjects with spastic extrinsic finger flexor muscles. Arch Phys Med Rehabil 1990 Oct;71(11):888–94.

Carey RG, Posavac EJ. Program evaluation of a physical medicine and rehabilitation unit: a new approach. Arch Phys Med Rehabil 1978 Jul;59(7):330–7.

Carr JH, Shepherd RB. A motor learning model for stroke rehabilitation. Physiotherapy 1989 Jul:75(7):372–80.

Carr JH, Shepherd RB, Nordholm L, Lynne D. Investigation of a new motor assessment scale for stroke patients. Phys Ther 1985 Feb;65(2):175–80.

Carter LT, Caruso JL, Languirand MA, Berard MA. Cognitive skill remediation in stroke and non-stroke elderly. Clinical Neuropsychology 1980;II(3):109–13.

Carter LT, Howard BE, O'Neil WA. Effectiveness of cognitive skill remediation in acute stroke patients. Am J Occup Ther 1983 May;37(5):320–6.

Chan F, Lynch R, Dial J, Wong D, Kates D. Applications of McCarron-Dial System in vocational evaluation: an overview of its operational framework and empirical findings. Vocational Eval and Work Adjustment Bull 1993:26(2):57–65.

Charness A. Stroke/head injury: a guide to functional outcomes in physical therapy management. Rockville (MD): Aspen Publishers; 1986.

Chen MY, Ott DJ, Peele VN, Gelfand DW. Oropharynx in patients with cerebrovascular disease: evaluation with videofluoroscopy. Radiology 1990 Sep;176(3):641–3.

Chenelly S. In: Dittmer S, editor. Rehabilitation nursing: process and application. St. Louis (MO): CV Mosby; 1989.

Clagett GP, Anderson FA, Levine MN, Salzman EW, Wheeler HB. Prevention of venous thromboembolism. Chest 1992 October;102(4):(Suppl) 391S–407S.

Clarke M, Kadhom HM. The nursing prevention of pressure sores in hospital and community patients. J Adv Nurs 1988 May;13(3):365–73.

Collen FM, Wade DT, Robb GF, Bradshaw CM. The Rivermead Mobility Index: a further development of the Rivermead Motor Assessment. Int Disabil Stud 1991;13:50–4.

Collin C, Wade D. Assessing motor impairment after stroke: a pilot reliability study. J Neurol Neurosurg Psychiatry 1990 Jul;53(7):576–9.

Connolly SJ, Laupacis A, Gent M, Roberts RS, Cairns JA, Joyner C. Canadian Atrial Fibrillation Anticoagulant (CAFA) Study. J Am Coll Cardiol 1991;18:349–55.

Cooper R, Sempos C, Hsieh SC, Kover MG. Slowdown in the decline of stroke mortality in the United States, 1978-1986. Stroke 1990;21:1274–9.

Corcoran PJ, Jebsen RH, Brengelmann GL, Simons BC. Effects of plastic and metal leg braces on speed and energy cost of hemiparetic ambulation. Arch Phys Med Rehabil 1970 Feb;51(2):69–77.

Coslett HB, Heilman KM. Male sexual function. Impairment after right hemisphere stroke. Arch Neurol 1986 Oct;43(10):1036–9.

Cote R, Battista RN, Wolfson C, Boucher J, Adam J, Hachinski V. The Canadian Neurological Scale: validation and reliability assessment. Neurology 1989 May;39:638–43.

Cote R, Hachinski VC, Shurvell BL, Norris JW, Wolfson C. The Canadian Neurological Scale: a preliminary study in acute stroke. Stroke 1986;17:731–7.

Cozean CD, Pease WS, Hubbell SL. Biofeedback and functional electrical stimulation in stroke rehabilitation. Arch Phys Med Rehabil 1988;69:401–5.

Crowe NM, Athelestan GT. Functional assessment in rehabilitation: systematic approach to diagnosis and goal setting. Arch Phys Med Rehabil 1981;62:229–305.

Culebras A. Neuroanatomic and neurologic correlates of sleep disturbances. Neurology 1992 Jul;42(Suppl 6):19–27.

Cushman LA. Secondary neuropsychiatric complications in stroke: implications for acute care. Arch Phys Med Rehabil 1988 Oct;69(10):877–9.

Davis G, Wilcox J. Adult aphasia rehabilitation: Applied pragmatics. San Diego (CA): College Hill; 1985.

DeJong G, Branch LG. Predicting the stroke patient's ability to live independently. Stroke 1982 Sep-Oct;13(5):648–55.

Demeurisse G, Demol O, Robaye E. Motor evaluation in vascular hemiplegia. Eur Neurol 1980;19(6):382–9.

De Weerdt W, Harrison M. Measuring recovery of arm-hand function in stroke patients: a comparison of the Brunnstrom-Fugl-Meyer test and the action research arm test. Physiother Can 1985;37(2):65–70.

Denes G, Semenza C, Stoppa E, Lis A. Unilateral spatial neglect and recovery from hemiplegia: a follow-up study. Brain 1982 Sep;105(Pt 3):543–52.

Depression Guideline Panel. Depression in primary care, Vol. 2; Treatment of major depression. Clinical practice guideline no. 5 (AHCPR Publication no. 93-0551). Rockville (MD): Agency for Health Care Policy and Research; 1993.

Dettmann MA, Linder MT, Sepic SB. Relationships among walking performance, postural stability, and functional assessments of the hemiplegic patient. Am J Phys Med 1987 Apr;66(2):77–90.

DeVincenzo DK, Watkins S. Accidental falls in a rehabilitation setting. Rehabil Nurs 1987 Sep-Oct;12(5):248–52.

Dickstein R, Hocherman S, Pillar T, Shaham R. Stroke rehabilitation. Three exercise therapy approaches. Phys Ther 1986 Aug;66(8):1233–8.

DiIorio C, Price M. Swallowing: an assessment guide. Am J Nurs 1990 Jul:38–46.

Diller L, Weinberg J. Evidence for accident-prone behavior in hemiplegic patients. Arch Phys Med Rehabil 1970 Jun;51(6):358–63.

Diller L, Weinberg J. Response styles in perceptual retraining. In: Gordon WA, editor. Advances in stroke rehabilitation. Boston (MA): Andover Medical Pub; 1993. p. 162–82.

Dombovy ML. Rehabilitation and the course of recovery after stroke. In: Whisnant J, editor. Stroke: populations, cohorts, and clinical trials. Oxford; Boston: Butterworth-Heinemann; 1993.

Dombovy ML, Basford JR, Whisnant JP, Bergstralh EJ. Disability and use of rehabilitation services following stroke in Rochester, Minnesota, 1975-1979. Stroke 1987 Sep-Oct;18(5):830–6.

Dombovy ML, Sandok BA, Basford JR. Rehabilitation for stroke: a review. Stroke 1986 May-Jun;17(3):363–9.

Doolittle ND. The experience of recovery following lacunar stroke. Rehabil Nurs 1992;17(3):122–5.

Downhill JE, Robinson RG. Longitudinal assessment of depression and cognitive impairment following stroke. J Nerv Ment Dis 1994 Aug;182(8):425–31.

Drummond A. Leisure activity after stroke. Int Disabil Stud 1990;12(4):157–60.

Duke University Center for the Study of Aging and Human Development. Multidimensional functional assessment: the OARS methodology. Durham (NC): Duke University; 1978.

Duncan PW. Contemporary management of motor control problems: proceedings of the II Step Conference. Alexandria (VA): Foundation for Physical Therapy; 1992. Chapter 21, Stroke: physical therapy assessment and treatment.

Duncan PW, Chandler J, Studenski S, Hughes M, Prescott B. How do physiological components of balance affect mobility in older men? Arch Phys Med Rehabil 1993 Dec;74(74):1343–9.

Duncan PW, Propst M, Nelson SG. Reliability of the Fugl-Meyer assessment of sensorimotor recovery following cerebrovascular accident. Phys Ther 1983 Oct;63(10):1606–10.

Dyken ML, Wolf PA, Barnett HJM, Bergan JJ, Hass WK, Kannel WB, Kuller L, Kurtzke JF, Sundt TM. Risk factors in stroke: a statement for physicians by the Subcommittee on Risk Factors and Stroke Council. Stroke 1984;15:1105–11.

Eastwood MR, Rifat SL, Nobbs H, Ruderman J. Mood disorders following cerebrovascular accident. Br J Psychiatry 1989;154:195–200.

Ebrahim S, Barer KD, Nouri F. Affective illness after stroke. Br J Psychiatry 1987;151:52–60.

Emick-Herring B, Wood P. A team approach to neurologically based swallowing disorders. Rehabil Nurs 1990 May-Jun;15(3):126–32.

Engel BT, Burgio LD, McCormick KA, et al. Behavioral treatment of incontinence in the long-term care setting. J Am Geriatr Soc 1990 38(3):361–3.

Epstein NB, Baldwin LM, Bishop DS. The McMaster Family Assessment Device. J Marital Fam Ther 1983 Apr;9(2):171–80.

Ernst E. A review of stroke rehabilitation and physiotherapy. Stroke 1990 Jul;21(7):1081–4.

European Carotid Surgery Trialists Collaborative Group. MRC European carotid surgery trial: interim results for symptomatic patients with severe (79-99%) or with mild (0-29%) carotid stenosis. Lancet 1991;337:1235–43.

Evans RL. Caregiver compliance and feelings of burden in poststroke home care. Psychol Rep 1986;59:1013–14.

Evans RL, Bishop DS, Dusley RT. Providing care to persons with disability: effect on family caregivers. Am J Phys Med Rehabil 1992;71(3)140–4.

Evans RL, Bishop DS, Haselkorn JK. Factors predicting satisfactory home care after stroke. Arch Phys Med Rehabil 1991 Feb;72:144–7.

Evans RL, Bishop DS, Matlock AL, Stranahan S, Smith GG, Halar EM. Family interaction and treatment adherence after stroke. Arch Phys Med Rehabil 1987a Aug;68(8):513–7.

Evans RL, Bishop DS, Matlock AL, Stranahan S, Noonan C. Predicting poststroke family function: a continuing dilemma. Psychol Rep 1987b;60:691–5.

Evans RL, Hendricks RD, Lawrence-Umlauf KV, Bishop DS. Timing of social work intervention and medical patients' length of hospital stay. Health Soc Work 1989 Nov:277–82.

Evans RL, Matlock AL, Bishop DS, Stranahan S, Pederson C. Family intervention after stroke: does counseling or education help? Stroke 1988 Oct;19(10):1243–9.

Evans R, Noonan WC. Does caregiver anxiety influence adjustment to stroke? Arch Phys Med Rehab 1988;69:799.

Ezekowitz MD, Bridgers SE, James KE, Carliner NH, Colling CL, Gornick CC, Krause-Steinrauf H, Kurtzke JF, Nazarian SM, Radford MJ, et al. Warfarin in the prevention of stroke associated with nonrheumatic atrial fibrillation. N Engl J Med 1992;327:1406–12.

Feigenson JS, Gitlow HS, Greenberg SD. The disability oriented rehabilitation unit: a major factor influencing stroke outcome. Stroke 1979 Jan-Feb;10(1):5–8.

Feinstein AR. Clinimetrics. New Haven (CT): University Press; 1987.

Feldman DJ, Lee PR, Unterecker J, Lloyd K, Rusk HA, Toole A. A comparison of functionally orientated medical care and formal rehabilitation in the management of patients with hemiplegia due to cerebrovascular disease. J Chronic Dis 1962;15:197–310.

Ferrucci L, Bandinelli S, Guralnik JM, Lamponi M, Bertini C, Falchini M, Baroni A. Recovery of functional status after stroke: a postrehabilitation follow-up study. Stroke 1993;24:200–5.

Fiatarone MA, Marks EC, Ryan ND, Meredith CN, Lipsitz LA, Evans WJ. High-intensity strength training in nonagenarians. Effects on skeletal muscle. JAMA 1990 Jun 13;263(22):3029–34.

Folstein MF, Folstein SE, McHugh PR. Mini-mental state: a practical method for grading the cognitive state of patients for the clinician. J Psychiatr Res 1975 Nov;12(3):189–98.

Foulkes MA, Wolf PA, Price TR, Mohr JP, Hier DB. The stroke data bank: design, methods, and baseline characteristics. Stroke 1988 May;19(5):547–54.

Friedland J, McColl M. Social support and psychosocial dysfunction after stroke: buffering effects in a community sample. Arch Phys Med Rehabil 1987 Aug;68(8):475–80.

Friedland JF, McColl M. Social support intervention after stroke: results of a randomized trial. Arch Phys Med Rehabil 1992 Jun;73(6):573–81.

Fristad MA. A comparison of the McMaster and Circumplex family assessment instruments. J Marital Fam Ther 1989;15(3):259–69.

Fugl-Meyer AR, Jaasko L, Leyman I, Olsson S, Steglind S. The post stroke hemiplegic patient. I. A method for evaluation of physical performance. Scand J Rehabil Med 1975;7:13–31.

Fullerton KJ, McSherry D, Stout RW. Albert's test: a neglected test of perceptual neglect. Lancet 1986 Feb 22;1(8478):430–2.

Galski T, Bruno RL, Zorowitz R, Walker J. Predicting length of stay, functional outcome, and aftercare in the rehabilitation of stroke patients. The dominant role of higher-order cognition. Stroke 1993 Dec;24(12):1794–800.

Garlinghouse NM. Sexuality of male cerebral vascular accident victims. Sex and Disabil 1987 Summer;8(2):67–72.

Garraway WM, Akhtar AJ, Hockey L, Prescott RJ. Management of acute stroke in the elderly: follow-up of a controlled trial. BMJ 1980 Sep 27;281:827–9.

Garraway WM, Akhtar AJ, Prescott RJ, Hockey L. Management of acute stroke in the elderly: preliminary results of a controlled trial. BMJ 1980 Apr 12;280(6220):1040–3.

Garraway WM, Akhtar AJ, Smith DL, Smith ME. The triage of stroke rehabilitation. J Epidemiol Community Health 1981 Mar;35(1):39–44.

Garraway WM, Walton MS, Akhtar AJ, Prescott RJ. The use of health and social services in the management of stroke in the community: results from a controlled trial. Age Ageing 1981 May;10(2):95–104.

Garraway WM, Whisnant JP, Drury I. The changing pattern of survival following stroke. Stroke 1983;14:699–703.

Gelber DA, Good DC, Laven LJ, Verhulst SJ. Causes of urinary incontinence after acute hemispheric stroke. Stroke 1993;24(3):378–82.

Gerson LW. The incidence of pressure sores in active treatment hospitals. Int J Nurs Stud 1975;12(4):201–4.

Gillum RF. Strokes in blacks. Stroke 1988;19:1–6.

Glanz M, Klawansky S, Stason W, Berkey C, Shah N, Phan H, Chalmers TC. Biofeedback therapy in post-stroke rehabilitation. A meta-analysis of the randomized control trials. Unpublished paper, 1994a.

Glanz M, Klawansky S, Stason W, Berkey C, Shah N, Phan H, Chalmers T. Functional electrical stimulation in post-stroke rehabilitation: a meta-analysis of randomized control trials. Unpublished paper, 1994b.

Glass TA, Matchar DB, Belyea M, Feussner JB. Impact of social support on outcome in first stroke. Stroke 1993;24:64–70.

Glasser L. Effects of isokinetic training on the rate of movement during ambulation in hemiparetic patients. Phys Ther 1986 May;66(5):673–6.

Goldman HH, Skodol AE, Lave TR. Revising Axis V for DSM-IV: a review of measures of social functioning. Am J Psychiatry 1992 Sep;149(9):1148–56.

Goldstein LB. Basic and clinical studies of pharmacologic effects on recovery from brain injury. J Neural Transplant Plast 1993 Jul-Sep;4(3):175–92.

Goldstein LB, Bertels C, Davis JN. Interrater reliability of the NIH stroke scale. Arch Neurol 1989 Jun;46(6):660–2.

Goodglass H, Kaplan E. The assessment of aphasia and related disorders. Philadelphia: Lee and Febiger; 1972. Chapter 4, Test procedures and rationale. Manual for the BDAE.

Goodglass H, Kaplan E. Boston Diagnostic Aphasia Examination (BDAE). Philadelphia: Lea and Febiger; 1983.

Gordon J. Assumptions underlying physical therapy intervention: theoretical and historical perspectives. In: Carr J, Shepherd RB, Gordon J, et al., editors. Movement science foundations for physical therapy in rehabilitation. Rockville (MD): Aspen Publishers Inc.; 1987. p. 1–30.

Gordon WA. Treatment of affective deficits in stroke rehabilitation. Final report, National Institutes of Health; NS 24608; 1992.

Gordon WA, Diller L. Stroke: coping with a cognitive deficit. In: Burish TG, Bradley LA, editors. Coping with chronic disease. New York: Academic Press; 1983.

Gordon WA, Hibbard MR, Egelko S, Diller L, Shaver MS, Lieberman A, Ragnarsson K. Perceptual remediation in patients with right brain damage: a comprehensive program. Arch Phys Med Rehabil 1985 Jun;66(6):353–94.

Gordon WA, Hibbard MR, Egelko S, Riley E, Simon D, Ross E, Leiberman A. Issues in the diagnosis of post stroke depression. Rehab Psychol 1991;36:71–87.

Granger CV. A conceptual model for functional assessment. In: Granger CV, Gresham GE, editors. Functional assessment in rehabilitation medicine. Baltimore: Williams & Wilkins; 1984. p. 14–25.

Granger CV, Albrecht GL, Hamilton BB. Outcome of comprehensive medical rehabilitation: measurement by PULSES profile and the Barthel Index. Arch Phys Med Rehabil 1979 Apr;60(4):145–54.

Granger CV, Dewis LS, Peters NC, Sherwood CC, Barrett JE. Stroke rehabilitation: analysis of repeated Barthel Index measures. Arch Phys Med Rehabil 1979 Jan;60(1):14–7.

Granger CV, Hamilton BB. Measurement of stroke rehabilitation outcome in the 1980s. Stroke 1990 Sep;21(Suppl II):II46–7.

Granger CV, Hamilton BB. UDS Report: The uniform data system for medical rehabilitation report on the first admissions for 1990. Am J Phys Med Rehabil 1992;71:108–13.

Granger CV, Hamilton BB, Keith RA, Zielezny M, Sherwin FS. Advances in functional assessment for medical rehabilitation. Top Geriatr Rehabil 1986;1(3):59–74.

Granger CV, Hamilton BB, Sherwin FS. Guide for the use of the uniform data set for medical rehabilitation. Buffalo General Hospital, Uniform Data System for Medical Rehabilitation Project Office. New York; 1986.

Greenberg S, Fowler RS Jr. Kinesthetic biofeedback: a treatment modality for elbow range of motion in hemiplegia. Am J Occup Ther 1980 Nov;34(11):738–43.

Gresham GE, Phillips TF, Labi ML. ADL status in stroke: relative merits of three standard indexes. Arch Phys Med Rehabil 1980 Aug;61(8):355–8.

Gresham GE, Phillips TF, Wolf PA, McNamara PM, Kannel WB, Dawber TR. Epidemiologic profile of long-term stroke disability: the Framingham Study. Arch Phys Med Rehabil 1979;60(11):487–91.

Gross JC. Bladder dysfunction after a stroke—it's not always inevitable. J Gerontol Nurs 1990 Apr;16(4):20–5.

Guide for the uniform data set for medical rehabilitation (Adult FIM), version 4.0. Buffalo (NY) 14214: State University of New York at Buffalo; 1993.

Gwyther LP, George LK. Caregivers of dementia patients: complex determinants of well-being and burden. Gerontologist 1986;26:245–7.

Halstead L. Team care in chronic illness: a critical review of the literature of the past 25 years. Arch Phys Med Rehabil 1976;57:507–11.

Hamilton M. Development of a rating scale for primary depressive illness. Br J Soc Clin Psychol 1967;6:278–96.

Hamilton M. A rating scale for depression. J Neurol Neurosurg Psychiatry 1960;23:56–62.

Hamilton BB, Granger CV, Sherwin FS, Zielezny M, Tashman JS. A uniform national data system for medical rehabilitation. In: Fuhrer MJ, editor. Rehabilitation outcomes: analysis and measurement. Baltimore: Brookes; 1987. p. 137–147.

Hamilton BB, Laughlin JA, Granger CV, Kayton RM. Interrater agreement of the seven level functional independence measure (FIM). Arch Phys Med Rehabil 1991;72:790.

Hamrin E. II. Early activation in stroke: does it make a difference? Scand J Rehabil Med 1982a;14(3):101–9.

Hamrin E. III. One year after stroke: a follow-up of an experimental study. Scand J Rehabil Med 1982b;14(3):111–6.

Harmsen P, Tsipogianni A, Wilhelmsen L. Stroke incidence rates were unchanged, while fatality rates declined, during 1971-1987 in Goteborg, Sweden. Stroke 1992;23:1410–15.

Hartman J, Landau WM. Comparison of formal language therapy with supportive counseling for aphasia due to acute vascular accident. Arch Neurol 1987;44:646–9.

Harvey RF, Jellinek HM. Functional performance assessment: a program approach. Arch Phys Med Rehabil 1981;62:456–61.

Hayes SH, Carroll SR. Early intervention care in the acute stroke patient. Arch Phys Med Rehabil 1986 May;67(5):319–21.

Helm-Estabrooks N, Emery P, Albert ML. Treatment of aphasic perseveration (TAP) program. A new approach to aphasia therapy. Arch Neurol 1987;44:1253–5.

Helm-Estabrooks N, Fitzpatrick P, Barresi B. Visual action therapy for global aphasia. J Speech Hear Disord 1982:44:385–9.

Hertanu JS, Demopoulos JT, Yang WC, Calhoun WF, Fenigstein HA. Stroke rehabilitation: correlation and prognostic value of computerized tomography and sequential functional assessments. Arch Phys Med Rehabil 1984 Sep;65(9):505–8.

Hibbard MR, Gordon WA. The comprehensive psychological assessment of individuals with stroke. J Neurol Rehabil 1992;2(4):9–20.

Hibbard MR, Gordon WA, Stein DN, et al. Awareness of disability in patients following stroke. Rehabil Psychol 1992;37:103–19.

Hibbard MR, Gordon WA, Stein P, Grober S, Sliwinski M. A multimodal approach to the diagnosis of post stroke depression. In: Gordon WA, editor. Advances in stroke rehabilitation. Boston: Andover Publishers; 1993.

Hier DB, Edelstein G. Deriving clinical prediction rules from stroke outcome research. Stroke 1991 Nov;22(11):1431–6.

Hier DB, Mondlock J, Caplan LR. Behavioral abnormalities after right hemisphere stroke. Neurology 1983 Mar;33(3):337–44.

Hocherman S, Dickstein R, Pillar T. Platform training and postural stability in hemiplegia. Arch Phys Med Rehabil 1984 Oct;65(10):588–92.

Holbrook M, Skilbeck CE. An activities index for use with stroke patients. Age Ageing 1983 May;12(2):166–70.

Holland A. Pragmatic aspects of intervention in aphasia. J Neurolinguistics 1991;6:197–211.

Holland AL. The usefulness of treatment for aphasia: a serendipitous study. In: Brookshire RH, editor. Proceedings of the conference on clinical aphasiology. Minneapolis: BRK Publishers; 1980. p. 240–7.

Horner J, Massey EW. Silent aspiration following stroke. Neurology 1988 Feb;38(2):317–9.

Horner J, Massey EW, Riski JE, Lathrop DL, Chase KN. Aspiration following stroke: clinical correlates and outcome. Neurology 1988 Sep;38(9):1359–62.

House A, Dennis M, Hawton K, Warlow C. Methods of identifying mood disorders in stroke patients: experience in the Oxfordshire community stroke project. Age Ageing 1989 Nov;18(6):371–9.

House A, Dennis M, Morgridge L, Warlow C, Hawton K, Jones L. Mood disorders in the year after first stroke. Br J Psychiatry 1991;158:83–92.

House A, Dennis M, Warlow C, Hawton K, Molyneux A. The relationship between intellectual impairment and mood disorder in the first year after stroke. Psychol Med 1990;20:805–14.

Hurd WW, Pegram V, Nepomuceno C. Comparison of actual and simulated EMG biofeedback in the treatment of hemiplegic patients. Am J Phys Med 1980 Apr;59(2):73–82.

Hyams DE. Psychological factors in rehabilitation of the elderly. Gerontol Clin 1969;11:129–36.

Inaba M, Edberg E, Montgomery J, Gillis MK. Effectiveness of functional training, active exercise, and resistive exercise for patients with hemiplegia. Phys Ther 1973 Jan;53(1):28–35.

Indredavik B, Bakke F, Solberg R, Rokseth R, Haaheim LL, Holme I. Benefit of a stroke unit: a randomized controlled trial. Stroke 1991 Aug;22(8):1026–31.

Inglis J, Donald MW, Monga TN, Sproule M, Young MJ. Electromyographic biofeedback and physical therapy of the hemiplegic upper limb. Arch Phys Med Rehabil 1984 Dec;65(12):755–9.

Jette AM, Branch LG. The Framingham disability study. II. Physical disability among the aging. Am J Public Health 1981;71:1211–16.

Jimenez J, Morgan PP. Predicting improvement in stroke patients referred for inpatient rehabilitation. Can Med Assoc J 1979 Dec 8;121(11):1481–4.

John J. Failure of electrical myofeedback to augment the effects of physiotherapy in stroke. Int J Rehabil Res 1986;9(1):35–45.

Johnston K, Olson E. Application of Bobath principles for nursing care of the hemiplegic patient. ARN J 1980 Mar-Apr;5(2):8–11.

Jonas S. Anticoagulant therapy in cerebrovascular disease: review and meta analysis. Stroke 1988;19:1043–8.

Jongbloed L. Prediction of function after stroke: a critical review. Stroke 1986 Jul-Aug;17(4):765–76.

Jongbloed L, Morgan D. An investigation of involvement in leisure activities after a stroke. Am J Occup Ther 1991 May;45(5):420–7.

Jongbloed L, Stacey S, Brighton C. Stroke rehabilitation: sensorimotor integrative treatment versus functional treatment. Am J Occup Ther 1989 Jun;43(6):391–7.

Joslin B, Coyne A, Johson T, et al. Dementia and elder abuse: are caregivers victims or villains? Annual Sci Meeting Gerontol Soc of America; 1991.

Judge JO, Lindsey C, Underwood M, Winsemius D. Balance improvements in older women: effects of exercise training. Physical Ther 1993;723:254–65.

Kabacoff RI, Miller IW, Bishop DS, Epstein NB, Keitner GI. A psychometric study of the McMaster Family Assessment Device in psychiatric, medical, and nonclinical samples. J Fam Psychol 1990 Jun;3(4):431–9.

Kalliomaki JL, Markkanen TK, Mustonen VA. Sexual behavior after cerebral vascular accident. Fert & Ster 1961;12(2):156–8.

Kalra L, Dale P, Crome P. Improving stroke rehabilitation. Stroke 1993;24:1462–7.

Kase C, Wolf PA, Kelly-Hayes M, Kannel WB, Bachman DL, Linn RT, D'Agostino RB. Intellectual decline following stroke: the Framingham Study. Neurology 1987 Mar;37(Suppl I):119.

Katrak PH, Cole AMD, Poulos CJ, McCauley JCK. Objective assessment of spasticity, strength, and function with early exhibition of dantrolene sodium after cerebrovascular accident: a randomized double-blind study. Arch Phys Med Rehabil 1992 Jan;73:4–9.

Katz S, Ford AB, Moskowitz RW, Jackson BA, Jaffe MW. Studies of illness in the aged. The index of ADL: a standardized measure of biological and psychosocial function. JAMA 1963 Sep 21:914–9.

Katz RT, Golden RS, Butter J, Tepper D, Rothke S, Holmes J, Sahgal V. Driving safety after brain damage: follow-up of twenty-two patients with matched controls. Arch Phys Med Rehabil 1990 Feb;71:133–7.

Kaufman KL, Tarnowski KJ, Simonian SJ, Graves K. Assessing the readability of family assessment self-report measures. Psych Assess: J Consult & Clin Psychol 1991;3(4):697–700.

Keith RA, Granger CV, Hamilton BB, Sherwin FS. The functional independence measure: a new tool for rehabilitation. In: Eisenberg MG, Grzesiak RC, editors. Advances in clinical rehabilitation. Volume 1. New York: Springer-Verlag; 1987. p. 6–18.

Kelly-Hayes M, Jette AM, Wolf PA, D'Agostino RB, Odell PM. Functional limitations and disability among elders in the Framingham Study. Am J Public Health 1992 Jun;82:841–5.

Kelly-Hayes M, Wolf PA, Kannel WB, Sytkowski P, D'Agostino RB, Gresham GE. Factors influencing survival and need for institutionalization following stroke: the Framingham Study. Arch Phys Med Rehabil 1988 Jun;69(6):415–8.

Kelly-Hayes M, Wolf PA, Kase CS, Gresham GE, Kannel WB, D'Agostino RB. Time course of functional recovery after stroke: the Framingham Study. J Neurol Rehabil 1989;3(2):65–70.

Kertesz A. Western Aphasia Battery. New York: Grune & Stratton; 1982.

Kiernan RJ. The Neurobehavioral Cognitive Status Examination. Northern California Neuro Group; 1987.

Kiernan RJ, Mueller J, Langston JW, Van Dyke C. The Neurobehavioral Cognitive Status Examination: a brief but differentiated approach to cognitive assessment. Ann Intern Med 1987;107:481–5.

Kinsella G, Ford B. Acute recovery patterns in stroke patients: neuropsychological factors. Med J Aust 1980 Dec 13;2(12):663–6.

Kiyohara Y, Ueda K, Hasuo Y, Wada J, Kawano H, Kato I, Sinkawa A, Ohmura T, Iwamoto H, Omae T, Fujishima M. Incidence and prognosis of subarachnoid hemorrhage in a Japanese rural community. Stroke 1989;20:1150–5.

Kojima S, Omura T, Wakamatsu W, Kishi M, Yamazaki T, Iida M, Komachi Y. Prognosis and disability of stroke patients after 5 years in Akita, Japan. Stroke 1990;21:72–7.

Korner E, Flooh E, Reinhart B, Wolf R, Ott E, Krenn W, Lechner H. Sleep alteration in ischemic stroke. Eur Neurol 1986;25(2):104–10.

Kotila M, Waltimo O, Niemi ML, Loaksoner R, Lempinen M. The profile of recovery from stroke and factors influencing outcome. Stroke 1984 Nov-Dec;15(6):1039–44.

Kraft GH, Fitts SS, Hammond MC. Techniques to improve function of the arm and hand in chronic hemiplegia. Arch Phys Med Rehabil 1992 Mar;73(3):220–7.

Kramer M, German P, Anthony J, et al. Patterns of mental disorders among elderly residents of Eastern Baltimore. J Am Geriatr Soc 1985;33:236–45.

Krefting L, Krefting D. Leisure activities after a stroke: an ethnographic approach. Am J Occup Ther 1991 May;45(5):429–36.

Kumar R, Metter EJ, Mehta AJ, Chew T. Shoulder pain in hemiplegia. The role of exercise. Am J Phys Med Rehabil 1990 Aug;69(4):205–8.

Landi G, D'Angelo A, Boccardi E, Candelise L, Mannucci PM, Morabito A, Orazio EN. Venous thromboembolism in acute stroke. Prognostic importance of hypercoagulability. Arch Neurol 1992;49:279–83.

Langhorne P, Williams BO, Gilchrist W, Howie K. Do stroke units save lives? Lancet 1993 Aug;342:395–8.

Laupacis A, Albers G, Dunn M, Feinberg WM. Antithrombotic therapy in atrial fibrillation. Chest 1992;102:4265–335.

Lawton MP. Assessing the competence of older people. In: Kent D, Kastenbaum R, Sherwood S, editors. Research planning and action for the elderly. New York: Behavioral Publications; 1972.

Lawton MP. Instrumental Activities of Daily Living (IADL) Scale: original observer-rated version. Psychopharmacol Bull 1988a;24(4):785–7.

Lawton MP. Instrumental Activities of Daily Living (IADL) Scale: self-rated version. Psychopharmacol Bull 1988b;24(4):789–91.

Legh-Smith J, Wade DT, Hewer RL. Driving after a stroke. J R Soc Med 1986 Apr;79(4):200–3.

Lehmann JF, DeLateur BJ, Fowler RS Jr, Warren CG, Arnhold R, Schertzer G, Hurka R, Whitmore JJ, Masock AJ, Chambers KH. Stroke: Does rehabilitation affect outcome? Arch Phys Med Rehabil 1975 Sep;56(9):375–82.

Levin MF, Hui-Chan CW. Relief of hemiparetic spasticity by TENS is associated with improvement in reflex and voluntary motor functions. Electroencephalogr Clin Neurophysiol 1992 Apr;85(2):131–42.

Levine DN. Unawareness of visual and sensorimotor defects: hypothesis. Brain Cognition 1990;13:233.

Levy DE, Bates D, Caroona JJ, et al. Prognosis in non-traumatic coma. Ann Intern Med 1981;94:293–301.

Lichtenberg P, Barth J. Depression in elderly caregivers: a longitudinal study to test Lewinshen's model of depression. Med Psychother 1990;3:147–56.

Lichtenberg P, Christensen B, Metler L. The role of cognition and depression in functional recovery during geriatric rehabilitation. J Clin Exper Neuropsychotherapy 1993;15:108.

Lichtenberg PA, Gibbons TA. Geriatric rehabilitation and the older adult family caregiver. Neurorehabilitation 1992;3(1):62–71.

Lincoln NB, McGuirk E, Mulley GP, Lendrem W, Jones AC, Mitchell JR. Effectiveness of speech therapy for aphasic stroke patients. A randomised controlled trial. Lancet 1984 Jun 2;1(8388):1197–200.

Linden P, Siebens AA. Dysphagia: predicting laryngeal penetration. Arch Phys Med Rehabil 1983 Jun;64(6):281–4.

Lipkin DP, Scriven AJ, Crake T, Poole-Wilson PA. Six minute walking test for assessing exercise capacity in chronic heart failure. BMJ 1986;292:653–5.

Lipsey JR, Robinson RG, Pearlson GD, Rao K, Price TR. Nortriptyline treatment of post-stroke depression: a double-blind study. Lancet 1984 Feb 11;1(8372): 297–300.

Loewen SC, Anderson BA. Reliability of the modified Motor Assessment Scale and the Barthel index. Physical Therapy 1988;68:1077–81.

Logemann JA. A manual for the videofluoroscopic evaluation of swallowing. San Diego (CA): College Hill; 1986.

Logigian MK, Samuels MA, Falconer J, Zagar R. Clinical exercise trial for stroke patients. Arch Phys Med Rehabil 1983 Aug;64(8):364–7.

Lord JP, Hall K. Neuromuscular reeducation versus traditional programs for stroke rehabilitation. Arch Phys Med Rehabil 1986 Feb;67(2):88–91.

Lord SR, Clark RD, Webster IW. Postural stability and associated physiological factors in a population of aged persons. J Gerontol 1991 May;46(3):M69–76.

Louis Harris and Associates. The ICD survey of disabled Americans: bringing disabled Americans into the mainstream. A nationwide survey of 1,000 disabled people. Conducted for ICD-International Center for the Disabled, New York, New York in cooperation with the National Council on the Handicapped, Washington, DC; 1986.

Lovett S, Gallager D. Psychoeducational interventions for family caregivers. Behav Ther 1988;19:321–30.

Lundgren-Lindquist B, Aniansson A, Rundgren A. Functional studies in 79 year olds: walking performance and climbing capacity. Scand J Rehabil Med 1983;15:125–31.

MacKenzie CR, Charlson ME, Digioia D, et al. Can the Sickness Impact Profile measure change? An example of scale assessment. J Chronic Dis 1986;39:429–38.

MacNeil RD, Pringnitz TD. The role of therapeutic recreation in stroke rehabilitation. Ther Rec J 1982; Qu. 4:26–34.

Mahoney FI, Barthel DW. Functional evaluation: the Barthel Index. Maryland State Med J 1965;14:61–5.

Mandel AR, Nymark JR, Balmer SJ, Grinnell DM, O'Riain MD. Electromyographic versus rhythmic positional biofeedback in computerized gait retraining with stroke patients. Arch Phys Med Rehabil 1990 Aug;71(9):649–54.

Marsh EE III, Adams HP Jr, Biller J, Wasek P, Banwart K, Mitchell V, Woolson R. Use of antithrombotic drugs in the treatment of acute ischemic stroke: a survey of neurologists in practice in the United States. Neurology 1989;39:1631–4.

Marshall RS, Mohr JP. Current management of ischaemic stroke. J Neurol Neurosurg Psychiatry 1993;56:6–16.

Matchar DB, McCrory DC, Barnett HJM, Feussner JR. Medical treatment for stroke prevention. Ann Intern Med 1994 Jul 1;121(1):41–53.

Matsumoto N, Whisnant JP, Kurland LT, Okazaki H. Natural history of stroke in Rochester, Minnesota, 1955 through 1969: an extension of a previous study, 1945 through 1954. Stroke 1973;4:20–9.

Mayberg MR, Wilson SE, Yatsu F, et al. Carotid endarterectomy and prevention of cerebral ischaemia in symptomatic carotid stenosis. JAMA 1991;266:3289–94.

Maynard FM, Diokno AC. Urinary infection and complications during clean intermittent catheterization following spinal cord injury. J Urol 1984;132(5):943–6.

McCormick GP, Riffer DJ, Thompson MM. Coital positioning for stroke afflicted couples. Rehabil Nurs 1986 Mar-Apr;11(2):17–9.

McCormick KA, Scheve AAS, Leahy E. Nursing management of urinary incontinence in geriatric inpatients. Nurs Clin North Am 1988 23(1):231–64.

McFarlane AH, Norman GR, Streiner DL, Roy RG. The process of social stress: stable, reciprocal and mediating relationships. J Health Soc Behav 1983;24(2):160–73.

McGovern PG, Burke GL, Sprafka JM, Xue S, Folsom AR, Blackburn H. Trends in mortality, morbidity, and risk factor levels for stroke from 1960 through 1990. JAMA 1992 Aug 12;268(6):753–9.

McHorney CA, Ware JE, Rogers W, et al. The validity and relative precision of MOS short- and long-form health status scales and Dartmouth COOP charts: results from the Medical Outcomes Study. Med Care 1992;30(5 Suppl):MS253–65.

Meerwaldt JD. Spatial disorientation in right-hemisphere infarction: a study of the speed of recovery. J Neurol Neurosurg Psychiatry 1983;46:426–9.

Merletti R, Zelaschi F, Latella D, Galli M, Angeli S, Sessa MB. A control study of muscle force recovery in hemiparetic patients during treatment with functional electrical stimulation. Scand J Rehabil Med 1978;10(3):147–54.

Miller IW, Bishop DS, Epstein NB, Keitner GI. The McMaster Family assessment device: reliability and validity. J Marital and Fam Ther 1985 Oct;11(4):345–56.

Mion L, Gregor S, Chwirchak D, Paras W. Falls in the rehabilitation setting: incidence and characteristics. Rehabil Nurs 1989;14(1):17–22.

Mitchum CC, Handiges A, Berndt R. Model-guided treatment to improve written sentence production: a case study. Aphasiology 1993;7:71–110.

Mol VJ, Baker CA. Activity intolerance in the geriatric stroke patient. Rehabil Nurs 1991 Nov-Dec;16(6):337–43.

Monga TN, Lawson JS, Inglis J. Sexual dysfunction in stroke patients. Arch Phys Med Rehabil 1986 Jan;67(1):19–22.

Morris PLP, Robinson RG, Andrzejewski P, Samuels J, Price TR. Association of depression with 10-year poststroke mortality. Am J Psychiatry 1993;150:124–9.

Morris PLP, Robinson RG, Raphael B. Prevalence and course of post-stroke depression in hospitalized patients. Int J Psychiatry Med 1990;20:327–42.

Mulder T, Hulstijn W, van der Meer J. EMG feedback and the restoration of motor control. A controlled group study of 12 hemiparetic patients. Am J Phys Med 1986 Aug;65(4):173–88.

Mysiw WJ, Beegan JG, Gatens PF. Prospective cognitive assessment of stroke patients before inpatient rehabilitation. The relationship of the Neurobehavioral Cognitive Status Examination to functional improvement. Am J Phys Med Rehabil 1989 Aug;68(4):168–71.

Nadolsky J. An experimental trend in assessment. In: Smith C, Fry R, editors. National forum on issues in vocational assessment: the issue papers. Menomonie (WI): University of Wisconsin-Stout, Stout Vocational Rehabilitation Institute, Materials Development Center; 1985.

Nagi S. Disability concepts revisited: implications for prevention. In: Sussman MG, editor. Sociology and rehabilitation. Washington, DC: American Sociological Association; 1965. p. 100–13.

National Institute of Neurological Disorders and Stroke. Clinical advisory: carotid endarterectomy for patients with asymptomatic internal carotid artery stenosis. National Institutes of Health; Sep 28 1994.

National Association of Rehabilitation Facilities. Medical rehabilitation: what it is and where is it? Washington, DC; November 1988.

National Stroke Association Consensus Statement. Stroke: the first six hours, emergency evaluation and treatment. In: McDowell FH, editor. Stroke: clinical updates; 1993;2(1).

Niemi ML, Laaksonen R, Kotila M, Waltimo O. Quality of life 4 years after stroke. Stroke 1988 Sep;19(9):1101–7.

Norris JT, Gallager D, Wilson A, Winograd CH. Assessment of depression in geriatric medical outpatients: the validity of two screening measures. J Am Geriatr Soc 1987;35:989–95.

North American Symptomatic Carotid Endarterectomy Trial Collaborators. Beneficial effect of carotid endarterectomy in symptomatic patients with high-grade stenosis. N Engl J Med 1991;325:445–53.

Norton D, McLaren R, Exton-Smith AN. An investigation of geriatric nursing problems in the hospital. London: National Corporation for the Care of Old People; 1962.

Nouri FM, Tinson DJ, Lincoln NB. Cognitive ability and driving after stroke. International Disability Studies 1987;9:110–5.

Osmon DC, Smet IC, Winegarden B, Gandhavadi B. Neurobehavioral Cognitive Status Examination: its use with unilateral stroke patients in a rehabilitation setting. Arch Phys Med Rehabil 1992;73:414–8.

Oxfordshire Community Stroke Project. Incidence of stroke in Oxfordshire: first year's experience of a community stroke register. BMJ 1983;287:713–17.

Pain HSB, McLellan DL. The use of individualized booklets after stroke. Clin Rehabil 1990;4:265–72.

Palmer JB, DeChase AS. Rehabilitation of swallowing due to strokes. Phys Med Rehab Clin N Amer 1991;2:529–46.

Panel for the Prediction and Prevention of Pressure Ulcers in Adults 1992. Pressure ulcers in adults; prediction and prevention. Clinical practice guideline no. 3 (AHCPR publication no. 92-0047). Rockville (MD): Agency for Health Care Policy and Research.

Parikh RM, Eden DT, Price TR, Robinson RG. The sensitivity and specificity of the Center for Epidemiologic Studies Depression Scale in screening for post-stroke depression. Int J Psychiatry Med 1988;18(2):169–81.

Parikh RM, Robinson RG, Lipsey JR, Starkstein SE, Federoff JP, Price TE. The impact of post-stroke depression on recovery in activities of daily living over a two-year follow-up. Arch Neurol 1990;47:785–9.

Peterson P, Boysen G, Godtfredsen J, Andersen ED, Andersen B. Placebo-controlled, randomized trial of warfarin and aspirin for prevention of thromboembolic complications in chronic atrial fibrillation. Lancet 1989;1:175–8.

Phipps M. Total patient care: foundations and practice of adult health nursing rehabilitation. In: Harkness GG, Dincher J, editors. St. Louis (MO): Mosby Year Books; 1990.

Pizzamiglio L, Frasca R, Guariglia C, Incoccia C, Antonucci G. Effect of optokinetic stimulation in patients with visual neglect. Cortex 1990;26:535–40.

Poeck K, Huber W, Willmes K. Outcome of intensive language treatment in aphasia. J Speech Hear Disord 1989 Aug; 54:471–9.

Poole JL, Whitney SL, Hangeland N, Baker C. The effectiveness of inflatable pressure splints on motor function in stroke patients. Occup Ther J Res 1990 Nov-Dec;10(6):360–6.

Poole JL, Whitney SL. Motor assessment scale for stroke patients: concurrent validity and interrater reliability. Arch Phys Med Rehabil 1988 Mar;69 (3 Pt 1):195–7.

Poplingher AR, Pillar T. Hip fracture in stroke patients. Epidemiology and rehabilitation. Acta Orthop Scand 1985 Jun;56(3):226–7.

Porch B. Porch Index of Communicative Ability (PICA). Palo Alto (CA): Consulting Psychologists Press; 1981.

Portnow J, Kline T, Daly M, Peltier SM, Chin C, Miller JR. Multidisciplinary home rehabilitation: a practical model. Clinics in Geriatric Medicine 1991 Nov;7(4):695–706.

Prescott. Survey shows stroke to be one of the most expensive medical illnesses in the United States. Internal Medicine World Report 1994 June 15;9(12):1–5.

Radloff LS. The CES-D scale: a self-report depression scale for research in the general population. J Appl Psychol Meas 1977;1:385–401.

Rankin J. Cerebral vascular accidents in patients over the age of 60. Scott Med J 1957;2:200–15.

Rapport LJ, Webster JS, Fleming KL, Lindberg JW, Godlewski MC, Brhee JE, Abadee PS. Predictors of falls among right hemisphere stroke patients in the rehabilitation setting. Arch Phys Med Rehabil 1993;74:621–6.

Reding MJ, Orto LA, Winter SW, Fortuna IM, Di Ponte P, McDowell FH. Antidepressant therapy after stroke: a double-blind trial. Arch Neurol 1986 Aug;43(8):763–5.

Reding MJ, Winter SW, Hochrein SA, Simon HB, Thompson MM. Urinary incontinence after unilateral hemispheric stroke: a neurologic-epidemiologic perspective. J Neuro Rehabil 1987;1:25–30.

Robertson IH, Gray JM, Pentland B, Waite LJ. Microcomputer-based rehabilitation for unilateral left visual neglect: a randomized controlled trial. Arch Phys Med Rehabil 1990 Aug;71(9):663–8.

Robinson RG, Benson DF. Depression in aphasic patients: frequency, severity, and clinical-pathological correlations. Brain Lang 1981 Nov;14(2):282–91.

Robinson R, Bolduc GA, Kubos KL. Social functioning assessment in stroke patients. Arch Phys Med Rehabil 1985;66:496–500.

Robinson RG, Bolduc PL, Price TR. A two-year longitudinal study of post-stroke mood disorders: diagnosis and outcome at one and two years. Stroke 1987 Sep-Oct;18(5):837–43.

Robinson RG, Parikh RM, Lipsey JR, Starkstein SE, Price TR. Pathological laughing and crying following stroke: validation of a measurement scale and a double-blind study. Am J Psychiatry 1993;150:286–93.

Robinson RG, Price TR. Post-stroke depressive disorders: a follow-up study of 103 patients. Stroke 1982 Sep-Oct;13(5):635–41.

Robinson RG, Starr LB, Kubos KL, Price TR. A two-year longitudinal study of post-stroke mood disorders: findings during the initial evaluation. Stroke 1983 Sep-Oct;14(5):736–44.

Robinson RG, Starr LB, Lipsey JR, Rao K, Price TR. A two-year longitudinal study of poststroke mood disorders. In-hospital prognostic factors associated with six-month outcome. J Nerv Ment Dis 1985 Apr;173(4):221–6.

Robinson RG, Szetela B. Mood change following left hemispheric brain injury. Ann Neurol 1981;9:447–53.

Rosenbek D. The dysarthrias. In: Johns D, editor. Clinical management of neurogenic communicative disorders. Boston: Little Brown; 1985.

Rosow I, Breslau N. A Guttman health scale for the aged. J Gerontol 1966;21:556–9.

Rossi PW, Kheyfets S, Reding MJ. Fresnel prisms improve visual perception in stroke patients with homonymous hemianopsia or unilateral visual neglect. Neurology 1990 Oct;40(10):1597–9.

Roth EJ. The elderly stroke patient: principles and practices of rehabilitation management. Top Geriatr Rehabil 1988;3(4):27–61.

Roth EJ. Medical complications encountered in stroke rehabilitation. Phys Med Rehabil Clin N Amer 1991 Aug;2(3):563–78.

Roth EJ, Mueller K, Green D. Stroke rehabilitation outcome: impact of coronary artery disease. Stroke 1988 Jan;19(1):42–7.

Rothberg J. The rehabilitation team: future direction. Arch Phys Med Rehabil 1981;62:407–11.

Roy C. Shoulder pains in hemiplegia: a literature review. Clin Rehabil 1988;2:35–44.

Rubens AB. Caloric stimulation and unilateral visual neglect. Neurology 1985;35:1019–24.

Rubenstein LZ, Robbins AS, Josephson KR, Schulman BL, Osterweil D. The value of assessing falls in an elderly population: a randomized clinical trial. Ann Int Med 1990;131:308–16.

Rubenstein LZ, Schairer C, Wieland GD, Kane R. Systematic biases in functional status assessment of elderly adults: effects of different data sources. J Gerontol 1984 Nov;39(6):686–91.

Sabanthan K, Castleden CM, Mitchell CJ. The problem of bacteriuria with indwelling urethral catheterization. Age Ageing 1985;14(2):85–90.

Sacco RL, Wolf PA, Kannel WB, McNamara PM. Survival and recurrence following stroke. The Framingham Study. Stroke 1982 May-Jun;13(3):290–5.

Sandercock P, Willems H. Medical treatment of acute ischemic stroke. Lancet 1992;339:537–9.

Sarno MT. Functional Communication Profile (FCP). New York University Medical Center Monograph Department. New York: New York University; 1969.

Schenkenberg T, Bradford DC, Ajax ET. Line bisection and unilateral visual neglect in patients with neurologic impairment. Neurology 1980;30:509–17.

Schleenbaker RE, Mainous III AG. Electromyographic biofeedback for neuromuscular reeducation in the hemiplegic stroke patient: a meta-analysis. Arch Phys Med Rehabil 1993 Dec;74:1301–4.

Schnelle JF. Treatment of urinary incontinence in nursing home patients by prompted voiding. J Am Geriatr Soc 1990;38(3):356–60.

Schoening HA, Iversen IA. Numerical scoring of self-care status: a study of the Kenny self-care evaluation. Arch Phys Med Rehabil 1968 Apr;49(4):221–9.

Schubert DS, Burns R, Paras W, Sioson E. Decrease of depression during stroke and amputation rehabilitation. Gen Hosp Psychiatry 1992a Mar;14(2):135–41.

Schubert DS, Burns R, Paras W, Sioson E. Increase of medical hospital length of stay by depression in stroke and amputation patients: a pilot study. Psychother Psychosom 1992b;57(1-2):61–6.

Schubert DS, Taylor C, Lee S, Mentari A, Tamaklo W. Detection of depression in the stroke patient. Psychosomatics 1992a Summer; 33(3):290–4.

Schubert DS, Taylor C, Lee S, Mentari A, Tamaklo W. Physical consequences of depression in the stroke patient. Gen Hosp Psychiatry 1992b Jan;14(1):69–76.

Schuling J, de Haan R, Limburg M, Groenier KH. The Frenchay Activities Index: assessment of functional status in stroke patients. Stroke 1993 Aug;24(8):1173–7.

Schultz R, Uisintainer P, Williamson G. Psychiatric and physical morbidity effects of caregiving. J Gerontol Psych Sci 1990;45:181–91.

Schwamm LH, Van Dyke C, Keirnana RS, Merrin EL, Mueller J. The Neurobehavioral Cognitive Status Examination: comparison with the Cognitive Capacity Screening Examination and the Mini-Mental State Examination in a neurosurgical population. Ann Intern Med 1987;107:486–91.

Sedrat SM, Hecht JS. Urologic problems after stroke (part II). Stroke Clinical Updates 1993;4(Pt 2):21–4.

Shah S, Vanclay F, Cooper B. Improving the sensitivity of the Barthel Index for stroke rehabilitation. J Clin Epidemiol 1989;42(8):703–9.

Shank J (The National Center for Medical Rehabilitation Research). The role of therapeutic recreation in rehabilitation research. 1992 Mar 6.

Shewan C, Bandur D. Treatment of aphasia: a language-oriented approach. San Diego (CA): College Hill; 1982.

Shewan CM, Kertesz A. Effects of speech and language treatment on recovery from aphasia. Brain Lang 1984 Nov;23(2):272–99.

Shiavi RG, Champion SA, Freeman FR, Bugel HJ. Efficacy of myofeedback therapy in regaining control of lower extremity musculature following stroke. Am J Phys Med 1979 Aug;58(4):185–94.

Shinar D, Gross CR, Bronstein KS, et al. Reliability of the Activities of Daily Living Scale and its use in telephone interviews. Arch Phys Med Rehabil 1987;68:723–8.

Shinar D, Gross CR, Price TR, Banko M, Bolduc PL, Robinson RG. Screening for depression in stroke patients: the reliability and validity of the Center for Epidemiologic Studies Depression Scale. Stroke 1986 Mar-Apr;17(2):241–5.

Shinton R, Beevers G. Meta-analysis of relation between cigarette smoking and stroke. BMJ 1989 Mar 25;298(6676):789–94.

Shumway-Cook A, Anson D, Haller S. Postural sway biofeedback: its effect on reestablishing stance stability in hemiplegic patients. Arch Phys Med Rehabil 1988 Jun;69(6):395–400.

Silliman RA, Wagner EH, Fletcher RH. The social and functional consequences of stroke for elderly patients. Stroke 1987 Jan-Feb;18(1):200–3.

Silver FL, Norris JW, Lewis AJ, Hachinski VC. Early mortality following stroke: a prospective study. Stroke 1984;25:666.

Sivak M, Hill CS, Henson DL, Butler BP, Silber SM. Improved driving performance following perceptual training in persons with brain damage. Arch Phys Med Rehabil 1984;65:163–7.

Sivak M, Olsen PL, Kewman DG, Won H, Henson DL. Driving and perceptual/cognitive skills: behavioral consequences of brain damage. Arch Phys Med Rehabil 1981;62:476–83.

Sivenius J, Pyorala K, Heinonen OP, Salonen JT, Riekkinen P. The significance of intensity of rehabilitation of stroke—a controlled trial. Stroke 1985 Nov-Dec;16(6):928–31.

Sjogren K. Leisure after stroke. Int Rehabil Med 1982;4(2):80–7.

Sjogren K, Damber JE, Liliequist B. Sexuality after stroke with hemiplegia. I. Scand J Rehabil Med 1983;15:55–61.

Sjogren K, Fugl-Meyer AR. Adjustment to life after stroke with special reference to sexual intercourse and leisure. J Psychosom Res 1982;26(4):409–17.

Skilbeck CE, Wade DT, Hewer RL, Wood VA. Recovery after stroke. J Neurol Neurosurg Psychiatry 1983 Jan;46(1):5–8.

Smith DS, Goldenberg E, Ashburn A, Kinsella G, Sheikh K, Brennan PJ, Meade TW, Zutshi DW, Perry JD, Reeback JS. Remedial therapy after stroke: a randomised controlled trial. BMJ (Clin Res) 1981 Feb 14;282(6263):517–20.

Smith ME, Garraway WM, Smith DL, Akhtar AJ. Therapy impact on functional outcome in a controlled trial of stroke rehabilitation. Arch Phys Med Rehabil 1982 Jan;63(1):21–4.

Smolkin C, Cohen BS. Socioeconomic factors affecting the vocational success of stroke patients. Arch Phys Med Rehabil 1974 Jun;55:269–71.

Soderback I. The effectiveness of training intellectual functions in adults with acquired brain damage: an evaluation of occupational therapy methods. Scand J Rehabil Med 1988;20(2):47–56.

Springer L, Glindemann R, Huber W, Willmes K. How efficacious is PACE therapy when language systematic training is incorporated? Aphasiology 1991;5:391–9.

Starkstein SE, Robinson RG. Neuropsychiatric aspects of stroke. In: Coffey CE, Cummings JL, editors. Textbook of geriatric neuropsychiatry. Washington, DC: American Psychiatric Press, Inc.; 1994. p. 457–78.

Stephens M, Kinney J, Igrocki P. Stressors and well being among caregivers to older adults with dementia: the in-home versus nursing home experience. Gerontol 1991;31:217–23.

Stern PH, McDowell F, Miller JM, Robinson M. Effects of facilitation exercise techniques in stroke rehabilitation. Arch Phys Med Rehabil 1970 Sep;51(9):526–31.

Stevens RS, Ambler NR, Warren MD. A randomized controlled trial of a stroke rehabilitation ward. Age Ageing 1984 Mar;13(2):65–75.

Stineman MG, Granger CV. Epidemiology of stroke-related disability and rehabilitation outcome. Phys Med Rehabil Clin N Amer 1991 Aug;2(3):457–71.

Stone SP, Wilson B, Wroot A, Halligan PW, Lange LS, Marshall JC, Greenwood RJ. The assessment of visuo-spatial neglect after acute stroke. J Neurol Neurosurg Psychiatry 1991 Apr;54(4):345–50.

Strand T, Asplund K, Eriksson S, Hagg E, Lithner F, Wester PO. A non-intensive stroke unit reduces functional disability and the need for long-term hospitalization. Stroke 1985 Jan-Feb;16(1):29–34.

Stroke prevention in atrial fibrillation (SPAF) investigators. Stroke prevention in atrial fibrillation study final results. Circulation 1991;84:527–39.

Studenski S. Falls. 2nd ed. Calkins E, editor. The practice of geriatrics. Philadelphia: WB Saunders; 1992.

Studenski S, Duncan P, Chandler J. Postural responses and effector factors in persons with unexplained falls: results and methodologic issues. J Am Geriatr Soc 1991;39:229–34.

Sunderland A, Tinson DJ, Bradley EL, Fletcher D, Langton-Hewer R, Wade DT. Enhanced physical therapy improves recovery of arm function after stroke. A randomised controlled trial. J Neurol Neurosurg Psychiatry 1992 Jul;55(7):530–5.

Sunderland A, Tinson DJ, Bradley EL, Fletcher D, Langton-Hewer R, Wade DT. Enhanced physical therapy for arm function after stroke: a one year follow-up study. J Neurol Neurosurg Psychiatry 1994;57:856–8.

Susset V, Vobecky J, Black R. Disability outcome and self-assessment of disabled persons: an analysis of 506 cases. Arch Phys Med Rehabil 1979;60:50–6.

Takebe K, Kukulka CG, Narayan MG, Basmajian JV. Biofeedback treatment of foot drop after stroke compared with standard rehabilitation technique (Pt 2): effects on nerve conduction velocity and spasticity. Arch Phys Med Rehabil 1976 Jan;57(1):9–11.

Tangeman PT, Banaitis DA, Williams AK. Rehabilitation of chronic stroke patients: changes in functional performance. Arch Phys Med Rehabil 1990 Oct;71(11):876–80.

Tatemichi TK, Desmond DW, Paik M. Mini-Mental Status Exam as a screen for dementia after stroke. J Clin Exper Psych 1991;13:419.

Taub E, Miller NE, Novack TA, Cook EW, Fleming WC, Nepmuceno CS, Connell JS, Crago JE. Technique to improve chronic motor deficit after stroke. Arch Phys Med Rehabil 1993 April;74:347–54.

Taylor MM, Schaeffer JN, Blumenthal FS, Grisell JL. Perceptual training in patients with left hemiplegia. Arch Phys Med Rehabil 1971 Apr;52(4):163–9.

Teasdale G, Jennett B. Assessment of coma and impaired consciousness: a practical scalc. Lancet 1974;2:81–3.

Teasdale G, Knill-Jones R, Van der Sande J. Observer variability in assessing impaired consciousness and coma. J Neurol Neurosurg Psychiatry 1978;41:603–10.

Teasdale G, Murray G, Parker L, Jennett B. Adding up the Glasgow Coma Scale. Acta Neurochir 1979;28(Suppl):13–6.

Terent A. Stroke morbidity. In: Whisnant J, editor. Stroke: populations, cohorts, and clinical trials. Oxford; Boston: Butterworth-Heineman; 1993.

Therapeutics and Technology Assessment Subcommittee of the American Academy of Neurology. Assessment: melodic intonation therapy. Neurology 1994;44:566–8.

Thomas DF. Vocational Assessment Protocol (VAP). University of Wisconsin—Stout. Research and Training Center; 1990.

Tinetti M. Performance oriented assessment of mobility problems in elderly patients. JAGS 1986;34:119–25.

Tinetti ME, Baker DI, McAvay G, Claus EB, Garrett P, Gottschalk M, Koch ML, Trainor K, Horwitz RI. A multifactorial intervention to reduce the risk of falling among elderly people living in the community. N Engl J Med 1994 Sep 29;331(13):821–7.

Tinetti ME, Ginter SF. Identifying mobility dysfunctions in elderly patients: standard neuromuscular examination or direct assessment? JAMA 1988 Feb 26;259(8):1190–3.

Titus MN, Gall NG, Yerxa EJ, Roberson TA, Mack W. Correlation of perceptual performance and activities of daily living in stroke patients. Am J Occup Ther 1991 May;45(5):410–8.

Tombaugh TN, McIntyre NJ. The Mini-Mental Status Examination: a comprehensive review. J Am Geriatr Soc 1992;40:922–35.

Towle D, Lincoln NB, Mayfield LM. Service provision and functional independence in depressed stroke patients and the effect of social work intervention on these. J Neurol Neurosurg Psychiatry 1989 Apr;52(4):519–22.

Trombly CA, Thayer-Nason L, Bliss G, Girard CA, Lyrist LA, Brexa-Hooson A. The effectiveness of therapy in improving finger extension in stroke patients. Am J Occup Ther 1986 Sep;40(9):612–7.

Tucker MA, Davison JG, Ogle SJ. Day hospital rehabilitation—effectiveness and cost in the elderly: a randomised controlled trial. BMJ 1984;289:1209–12.

Urinary Incontinence Guideline Panel. Urinary incontinence in adults. Clinical practice guideline no. 2 (AHCPR publication no. 92-0038). Rockville (MD): Agency for Health Care Policy and Research; 1992.

van Swieten JC, Koudstaal PJ, Visser MC, Schouten HJ, van Gijn J. Interobserver agreement for the assessment of handicap in stroke patients. Stroke 1988 May;19(5):604–7.

van Zomeren AH, Brouwer WH, Minderhoud JM. Acquired brain damage and driving: a review. Arch Phys Med Rehabil 1987 Oct;68:697–705.

Veis SL, Logemann JA. Swallowing disorders in persons with cerebrovascular accident. Arch Phys Med Rehabil 1985 Jun;66(6):372–5.

Venn M, Taft L, Carpentier B, Applebaugh G. The influence of timing and suppository use on efficiency and effectiveness of bowel training after stroke. Rehabil Nurs 1992;17(3):116–20.

Viitanen M, Fugl-Meyer KS, Bernspang B, Fugl-Meyer AR. Life satisfaction in long-term survivors after stroke. Scand J Rehabil Med 1988;20:17–24.

Wade DT. In: Stevens A, Raftery J, editors. Health care needs assessment. The epidemiologically based needs assessment reviews. Volume 1. Oxford: Radcliffe Medical Press Ltd.; 1994. p. 111–255.

Wade DT. Measurement in neurological rehabilitation. Oxford: Oxford University Press; 1992.

Wade DT, Collen FM, Robb GF, Warlow CP. Physiotherapy intervention late after stroke and mobility. BMJ 1992 Mar 7;304(6827):609–13.

Wade DT, Collin C. The Barthel ADL Index: a standard measure of physical disability? Int Disabil Stud 1988;10(2):64–7.

Wade DT, Hewer RL. Functional abilities after stroke: measurement, natural history and prognosis. J Neurol Neurosurg Psychiatry 1987a Feb;50(2):177–82.

Wade DT, Hewer RL. Motor loss and swallowing difficulty after stroke: frequency, recovery, and prognosis. Acta Neurol Scand 1987b Jul;76(1):50–4.

Wade DT, Hewer RL, David RM, Enderby PM. Aphasia after stroke: natural history and associated deficits. J Neurol Neurosurg Psychiatry 1986 Jan;49(1):11–6.

Wade DT, Langton-Hewer R, Skilbeck CE, Bainton D, Burns-Cox C. Controlled trial of a home-care service for acute stroke patients. Lancet 1985 Feb 9;1(8424):323–6.

Wade DT, Legh-Smith J, Hewer RA. Depressed mood after stroke. A community study of its frequency. Br J Psychiatry 1987 Aug;151:200–5.

Wade DT, Legh-Smith J, Langton-Hewer R. Social activities after stroke: measurement and natural history using Frenchay Activities Index. Int Rehabil Med 1985;7:176–81.

Wade DT, Parker V, Langton-Hewer R. Memory disturbance after stroke: frequency and associated losses. Int Rehabil Med 1986;8(2):60–4.

Wade DT, Wood VA, Hewer RL. Recovery of cognitive function soon after stroke: a study of visual neglect, attention span and verbal recall. J Neurol Neurosurg Psychiatry 1988 Jan;51(1):10–3.

Ward G, Jamrozik K, Stewart-Wynne E. Incidence and outcome of cerebrovascular disease in Perth, Western Australia. Stroke 1988;19:1501–6.

Ware JE, Sherbourne CD. The MOS 36-item short-form health survey (SF-36): I. Conceptual framework and item selection. Med Care 1992 Jun;30(6):473–83.

Warlow C, Ogston D, Douglas AS. Deep venous thrombosis of the legs after strokes: Part 2—Natural history. BMJ 1976 May 15;1(6019):1181–3.

Warren M. Identification of visual scanning deficits in adults after cerebrovascular accident. Am J Occup Ther 1990 May;44(5):391–9.

Warren JW, Tenney JH, Hoopes JM, Muncie HL, Anthony WC. A prospective microbiologic study of bacteriuria in patients with chronic indwelling urethral catheters. J Infect Dis 1982;164(6):719–23.

Webb RJ, Lawson AL, Neal DE. Clean intermittent self-catheterization in 172 adults. Br J Urol 1990;65(1):20–3.

Webster JS, Rapport LJ, Godlewski MC, Abadee PS. Effect of attentional bias to right space on wheelchair mobility. J Clin Exper Neuropsychol 1994;16:129–37.

Weinberg J, Diller L, Gordon WA, Gerstman LJ, Lieberman A, Lakin P, Hodges G, Ezrachi O. Training sensory awareness and spatial organization in people with right brain damage. Arch Phys Med Rehabil 1979 Nov;60(11):491–6.

Weinberg J, Diller L, Gordon WA, Gerstman LJ, Lieberman A, Lakin P, Hodges G, Ezrachi O. Visual scanning training effect on reading-related tasks in acquired right brain damage. Arch Phys Med Rehabil 1977 Nov;58(11):479–86.

Weinberg J, Piasetsky E, Diller L, Gordon WA. Treating perceptual organization deficits in nonneglecting RBD stroke patients. J Clin Neuropsychol 1982;4:59–75.

Weinrich M, Steele R, Carlson G, Kleczewska M, Wertz R, Baker E. Processing of visual syntax by a globally aphasic patient. Brain Lang 1989;36:391–405.

Weissman MM, Sholomskas D, Pottengel M, Prusoff BA, Locke BZ. Assessing depressive symptoms in five psychiatric populations: a validity study. Am J Epidemiol 1977;106:203–14.

Wenniger WFMdB, Hagemand WJPM, Arrindell WA. Cross-national validity of dimensions of family functioning: first experiences with the Dutch version of the McMaster Family Assessment Device (FAD). Pers Indiv Diff 1993 Jun;14(6):769–81.

Wertz RT. Response to treatment in patients with apraxia of speech. In: McNeill M, Rosenbek J, Aronson, editors. Apraxia of speech: physiology, acoustics, linguistics, management. San Diego (CA): College-Hill; 1984.

Wertz RT, Collins MJ, Weiss D, Kurtzke JF, Friden T, Brookshire RH, Pierce J, Holtzapple P, Hubbard DJ, Porch BE, West JA, Davis L, Matovitch V, Morley GK, Resurrection E. Veterans Administration cooperative study on aphasia: a comparison of individual and group treatment. J Speech Hear Res 1981;24:580–94.

Wertz RT, Weiss DG, Aten JL, Brookshire RH, Garc:ia-Bu:nuel L, Holland AL, Kurtzke JF, LaPointe LL, Milianti FJ, Brannegan R, et al. Comparison of clinic, home, and deferred language treatment for aphasia. A Veterans Administration Cooperative Study. Arch Neurol 1986 Jul;43(7):653–8.

Whipple RH, Wolfson LI, Amerman P. The relationship of knee and ankle weakness to falls in nursing home residents: an isokinetic study. J Am Geriatr Soc 1987;35:13–20.

Whisnant JP, Fitzgibbons JP, Kurland LT, Sayre GP. Natural history of stroke in Rochester, Minnesota, 1945 through 1954. Stroke 1971;2:11–22.

Williams JBW. A structured interview guide for the Hamilton Depression Rating Scale. Arch Gen Psychiatry 1988;45:742–6.

Williams & Wilkins, editors. Guide to clinical preventive services: an assessment of the effectiveness of 169 interventions. Report of the U.S. Preventive Services Task Force. Washington, DC.; 1989.

Wilson B, Cockburn J, Halligan P. Development of a behavioral test of visuospatial neglect. Arch Phys Med Rehabil 1987 Feb; 68(2):98–102.

Winchester P, Montgomery J, Bowman B, Hislop H. Effects of feedback stimulation training and cyclical electrical stimulation on knee extension in hemiparetic patients. Phys Ther 1983 Jul; 63(7):1096–103.

Winstein CJ. Motor learning considerations in stroke rehabilitation. In: Duncan DW, Badke MB, editors. Stroke rehabilitation: recovery of motor control. Chicago: Year Book Mode Publishers, Inc.; 1987.

Winstein CJ, Gardner ER, McNeal DR, Barto PS, Nicholson DE. Standing balance training: effect on balance and locomotion in hemiparetic adults. Arch Phys Med Rehabil 1989 Oct;70(10):755–62.

Wityk RJ, Pessin MS, Kaplan RF, Caplan LR. Serial assessment of acute stroke using the NIH stroke scale. Stroke 1994 Feb;25(2):362–65.

Wolf PA, Abbott RD, Kannel WB. Atrial fibrillation: a major contributor to stroke in the elderly: the Framingham Study. Arch Intern Med 1987 Sep;147(9):1561–4.

Wolf PA, Cobb JL, D'Agostino RB. Epidemiology of stroke. In: Barnett HJM, Mohr JP, Stein BM, Yatsu FM, editors. Stroke: pathophysiology, diagnosis and management. 2nd ed. New York: Churchill Livingstone; 1992.

Wolf PA, D'Agostino RB, Odell P, Belanger AJ, Hodges D, Kannel WB. Alcohol consumption as a risk factor for stroke: the Framingham study. Am Neuro Assoc 1992:177.

Wolf PA, D'Agostino RB, O'Neal MA. Secular trends in stroke incidence and mortality. The Framingham Study. Stroke 1992 Nov;23(11):1551–5.

Wolf SL, LeCraw DE, Barton LA. Comparison of motor copy and targeted biofeedback training techniques for restitution of upper extremity function among patients with neurological disorders. Phys Ther 1989 Sept;69(9):719–35.

Wolf SL, LeCraw DE, Barton LA, Jann BB. Forced use of hemiplegic upper extremities to reverse the effect of learned nonuse among chronic stroke and head-injured patients. Exp Neurol 1989 May;104(2):125–32.

Wolfson L, Whipple R, Amerman P, Tobin JN. Gait assessment in the elderly: a gait abnormality rating scale and its relation to falls. J Gerontol 1990;45:M12–19.

Woo E, Proulx SM, Greenblatt DJ. Differential side effect profile of triazolam versus flurazepam in elderly patients undergoing rehabilitation therapy. J Clin Pharmacol 1991 Feb;31(2):168–73.

Wood-Dauphinee S, Shapiro S, Bass E, Fletcher C, Georges P, Hensby V, Mendelsohn B. A randomized trial of team care following stroke. Stroke 1984 Sep-Oct;15(5):864–72.

Wood-Dauphinee S, Williams J, Shapiro S. Examining outcome measures in a clinical study of stroke. Stroke 1990 May;21(5):731–9.

World Health Organization (WHO). International classification of impairments, disabilities, and handicaps (ICDIDH). Geneva; 1980.

World Health Organization. Stroke—1989. Recommendations on stroke prevention, diagnosis, and therapy: report of the WHO Task Force on Stroke and other Cerebrovascular Disorders. Stroke 1989 Oct;20(10):1407–31.

Yano K, Reed DM, MacLean CJ. Serum cholesterol and hemorrhagic stroke in Honolulu Heart Program. Stroke 1989;20:1460–4.

Yekutiel M, Guttman E. A controlled trial of the retraining of the sensory function of the hand in stroke patients. J of Neurol, Neurosurg, and Psychiatry 1993;56:241–4.

Yesavage JA, Brink TL, Rose TL, Lum O, Huang V, Adey M, Leirer VO. Development and validation of a geriatric depression screening scale: a preliminary report. J Psychiatr Res 1982-83;17(1):37–49.

Young JB, Forster A. The Bradford community stroke trial: eight week results. Clin Rehabil 1991;5:283–92.

Young JB, Forster A. The Bradford community stroke trial: results at six months. BMJ 1992 Apr;304:1085–9.

Zung WK. A self-rating depression scale. Arch Gen Psychiatry 1965 Jan;12:63–70.

Acronyms and Abbreviations

ADL	Activities of daily living
AHCPR	Agency for Health Care Policy and Research
BF	Biofeedback
CARF	Commission on Accreditation of Rehabilitation Facilities
CRRN	Certified rehabilitation registered nurse
CT	Computed tomography
CTRS	Certified therapeutic rehabilitation specialist
DVT	Deep vein thrombosis
FES	Functional electrical stimulation
HCFA	Health Care Financing Administration
IADL	Instrumental activities of daily living
JCAHO	Joint Commission on Accreditation of Healthcare Organizations
LCSW	Licensed clinical social worker
LOA	Leave of absence
MRI	Magnetic resonance imaging
NIH	National Institutes of Health
OT	Occupational therapy
OTR	Registered occupational therapist
PT	Physical therapy, physical therapist
PVR	Postvoid residual
RCT	Randomized controlled trial
SLP	Speech-language pathologist
WHO	World Health Organization

Glossary

Rehabilitation Professions

Medical Specialties

All physicians have completed 3 or 4 years of undergraduate college education and 4 years of medical school, and most have completed residency training in a specialty. During rehabilitation, the physician treats medical problems and often functions as the team leader. Physiatry and neurology are the medical specialties most commonly involved in rehabilitation. Geriatricians, internists, family physicians, and psychiatrists may also be involved.

Neurologist. Specializes in the diagnosis and treatment of diseases of the nervous system and has completed a minimum of 4 years of residency training after medical school.

Physiatrist. Specializes in physical medicine and rehabilitation and has completed a minimum of 4 years of residency training in physical medicine and rehabilitation after medical school.

Geriatrician. Specializes in internal medicine or family practice and has completed a minimum of 3 years of residency training after medical school, with additional training in the care of the elderly.

Occupational Therapy (OT)

Occupational therapists are primarily concerned with helping the patient learn to perform tasks and activities required by daily life.

Registered occupational therapist (OTR). Has completed 4 years of college and a 6-month supervised internship, and has been examined and certified by the American Occupational Therapy Certification Board (AOTCB).

Certified occupational therapist assistant (COTA). Has completed a 2-year or associate degree and a 12-week supervised internship, and has been examined and certified by the AOTCB.

Occupational therapy aide. Has been trained by the institution in which he or she works.

Physical Therapy (PT)

Physical therapists work with patients disabled by strokes to help them regain motor control, strength, physical conditioning and mobility, and return to independent living.

Physical therapist. Has completed at least 4 years of college, and many have completed a master's degree (6 years of higher education); all have successfully passed a State licensure examination.

Physical therapy assistant. Has completed 2 years of education after high school.

Physical therapy aide. Is trained by the institution in which he or she works.

Psychology

Psychologists assess the mental, cognitive, and emotional status of patients, work with the rehabilitation team to design treatment, and often provide treatment.

Clinical psychologist. Has completed a doctoral program in psychology and a 1-year internship.

Neuropsychologist. A specialized psychologist who emphasizes understanding and treatment of the cognitive, psychological, and behavioral problems that occur after damage to specific areas of the brain.

Recreational Therapy

Recreational therapists work with the rehabilitation team to assess functional and leisure abilities and to promote recovery through physical conditioning and leisure activities. Certification is offered by the National Council for Therapeutic Recreation Certification (NCTRC).

Certified therapeutic recreation specialist (CTRS). Has completed 4 years of college with a degree in therapeutic recreation (recreational therapy) or a degree in recreation with an emphasis in therapeutic recreation, has completed a supervised recreational therapy field-work placement of 36 hours, and has passed the national certification examination administered by NCTRC.

Certified therapeutic recreation assistant (CTRA). Has completed a 2-year or associate degree with a major in recreation or therapeutic recreation; a 10-week field placement may be required.

Rehabilitation Nursing

Rehabilitation nurses are specifically trained by experience, continuing education, or graduate education to provide nursing services to patients disabled by strokes or other chronic diseases, with the goals of restoring and maintaining health, function, independence, and quality of life for the patient and family, and the cost-effective use of resources.

Registered nurse (RN). Has completed a 2- or 3-year hospital-based program in nursing or a 2- or 4-year college program in nursing, and has successfully passed an examination by the State board of nursing.

Certified rehabilitation registered nurse (CRRN). A registered nurse (RN) with at least 2 years of experience in rehabilitation nursing who has been examined and certified by the Rehabilitation Nursing Certification Board.

Nurse practitioner. An RN who has met advanced educational and clinical practice requirements. A nurse practitioner conducts physical examinations, takes medical histories, orders and interprets laboratory tests and x-rays, diagnoses and treats common illnesses; and, in 43 States, prescribes medications.

Social Work

Social workers are integral members of the rehabilitation team with special responsibilities for working with patients and families to evaluate community and family resources, obtain necessary community services, and facilitate discharge planning. Social workers will also often provide counseling and education.

Licensed clinical social worker (LCSW). Typically, has completed 4 years of college and a 2-year master's program in social work (MSW) and has been licensed by a State examining board. Requirements vary by State.

Speech Therapy

Speech-language pathologists work with patients with aphasia, dysarthria, and dysphagia.

Speech-language pathologist (SLP). Has completed 4 years of college, a master's degree in speech-hearing-language pathology, 375 hours of supervised clinical observation, and a 36-week clinical fellowship. SLPs obtain a Certificate of Clinical Competence (CCC) from the American Speech-Language-Hearing Association (ASHA).

Dietitians

The dietitian assesses the nutritional status of the patient and provides diet therapy, counseling, or specialized nutritional supplements.

Registered dietitian. Has completed a baccalaureate degree granted by a U.S. regionally accredited college or university; has met current academic requirements as approved by the American Dietetic Association; has successfully completed the Registration Examination for Dietitians; and has accrued 75 hours of approved continuing education every 5 years.

General Terms in Stroke Rehabilitation

Activation. Stimulating the nervous system through encouraging the patient who has suffered a stroke to become mentally and physically active.

Activities of daily living (ADL). Basic daily activities such as eating, grooming, toileting, and dressing.

Acute care hospital. A hospital that is organized and staffed to provide care for patients with acute medical problems.

Acute rehabilitation. Term used by some sources to denote intense rehabilitation in an inpatient rehabilitation facility.

Ambulation. The act of walking.

Assessment. Determining the scope, importance, and value of a medical or psychological condition, social or environmental situation, or treatment.

Biofeedback. Use of visual or auditory feedback on the state of a physiologic function (such as heart rate) or the position of a part of the body (such as the arm or leg) with the purpose of helping the individual gain better control over the function or position.

Caregiver. A person who provides direct support for a disabled individual, usually in the home.

Comorbidity. One or more additional chronic diseases in an individual who has suffered a stroke, such as heart or lung disease.

Compensation. The ability of an individual with disabilities from stroke to perform a task (or tasks) either using the impaired limb with an adapted (different) approach or using the unaffected limb to perform the task; an approach to rehabilitation in which the patient is taught to adapt to and offset residual disabilities.

Comprehensive rehabilitation. Rehabilitation involving a full array of rehabilitation services and disciplines (physical therapy, occupational therapy, speech and language pathology, recreational therapy, mental health services, etc.).

Continence. The ability to control bodily functions, especially urinary bladder and bowel function.

Counseling. Supportive and educational interventions aimed at assisting the patient or family in identifying key issues and problem solving around them.

Deconditioning. The loss of cardiovascular or physical fitness as a result of inactivity.

Deficit. Loss of ability. In the case of a stroke, a loss of neurological function.

Disability. Reduced ability or lack of ability of an individual to perform an activity in daily life.

Family. Relatives or friends who live with or are close to the patient.

Forced use. Use of an impaired limb encouraged by restraining the unaffected limb and, hence, preventing it from taking over performance of required tasks.

Functional electrical stimulation. Bursts of electrical stimulation applied to the nerves or muscles affected by the stroke, with the goal of strengthening muscle contraction and improving motor control. Lower intensities (transcutaneous electrical nerve stimulation, or TENS) are also used for pain control.

Functional limitation. Reduced ability or lack of ability to perform an action or activity in the manner or within the range considered to be normal.

Gait symmetry. A normal walking pattern, in which the movements of one leg are mirrored by similar movements of the other leg.

Handicap. A disadvantage resulting from an impairment or disability that limits or prevents fulfillment of a role that is normal for the affected individual.

Impairment. The loss or abnormality of physical or psychological capacities.

Independent. Able to perform all usual functions without assistance or supervision.

Inpatient. An individual who is receiving care while being housed in a medical facility.

Institutionalization. Custodial care of a mentally or physically dependent individual in a long-term care facility.

Instrumental activities of daily living (IADL). Complex activities required for independent living, such as using a telephone, home management, cooking, use of public transportation, or financial management.

Intense rehabilitation. Generally interpreted to mean rehabilitation involving 3 or more hours of acute physical, occupational, psychological, or speech and language therapy per day, 5 or more days per week.

Interdisciplinary treatment. Treatment delivered to a patient by two or more medical or rehabilitative disciplines working collaboratively.

Medical stability. Maintaining a constant health status in the face of diseases that threaten to upset it.

Mobility. Ability to move freely.

Mobilization. The act of getting a patient to move in bed, sit up, stand, and eventually walk.

Monitoring. Repetitive checking of a patient's medical, neurological, and functional status.

Motor control. Ability to control movements of the body.

Nursing facility. A nursing home.

Orthoses. Mechanical devices which apply pressure to parts of the body in order to support, correct, or aid function.

Outpatient. A person receiving treatment in a hospital, clinic, or office without being hospitalized.

Pathology. The interruption of, or interference with, normal bodily processes or structures by a disease process.

Postacute care. Care delivered during convalescence after an acute illness.

Primary physician. The physician who is responsible for the care of a patient's general medical problems and for the coordination of required specialty care; this is usually an internist, family practitioner, general practitioner, pediatrician, or obstetrician, but may be from any specialty.

Prophylaxis. Treatments aimed at preventing disease.

Psychotherapy. Interventions aimed at changing basic mental functions in an individual or organizational or transactional patterns in families.

Range of motion exercises. Exercises during which joints are moved through their full degrees of flexion, extension, or rotation; range of motion exercise is "active" if the patient provides the power needed to move the joint or "passive" if the therapist provides the power.

Rehabilitation. Restoration of the disabled person to self-sufficiency or maximal possible functional independence.

Rehabilitation hospital. A freestanding hospital that is organized and staffed to provide intense and comprehensive inpatient rehabilitation.

Rehabilitation unit. A distinct part of an acute care hospital that is organized and staffed to provide intense and comprehensive inpatient rehabilitation.

Reliability, interobserver. A characteristic of assessment procedures or instruments that refers to the ability of different observers to obtain the same results in the same patient, provided that there has been no change in the patient's condition.

Reliability, test-retest. A characteristic of assessment procedures or instruments that refers to the ability to obtain the same result at different points in time in a patient whose condition remains unchanged.

Remediation. Approaches to rehabilitation that attempt to reduce the severity of neurological deficits.

Screening. Examinations aimed at detecting medical conditions early in their course or before they become symptomatic, often with the purpose of implementing treatment that will prevent or ameliorate the problem.

Self-care. Providing care for oneself, e.g., by performing one's own basic activities of daily living.

Sensibility. The characteristics of an assessment procedure or instrument that refer to its reasonableness, importance, and ease of use.

Sensitivity. The ability of an assessment procedure or instrument to detect clinically meaningful change.

Stroke unit. A distinct part of an acute care hospital that is organized and staffed explicitly to provide care for patients with strokes.

Subacute rehabilitation. A term used by some sources to refer to rehabilitation programs provided in nursing facilities.

Medical and Neurological Terms

Agraphia. Inability to express one's thoughts in writing.

Alexia. Inability to understand written language.

Aneurysm. A sac created by expansion of an artery, vein, or the heart.

Angiography. A method of visualizing blood vessels by introducing a radiographic solution.

Anterior. The front of the body or an organ.

Aphasia. The loss of ability to communicate orally, through signs, or in writing, or the inability to understand such communications; the loss of language usage ability.

Apraxia. A disorder of learned movement unexplained by deficits in strength, coordination, sensation, or comprehension.

Aspiration. The act of inhaling solid or liquid materials into the lungs.

Astereognosis. The inability to recognize or characterize objects by touch.

Ataxia. A disorder in which muscles fail to move in a coordinated fashion.

Atrial fibrillation. Rapid, irregular contraction of the atria of the heart that produces an irregular and often rapid ventricular rate.

Cardiac arrhythmia. Irregular or abnormally slow or rapid beating of the heart.

Cardiovascular. Pertaining to the heart and blood vessels.

Carotid artery. A major artery in the neck that supplies blood to the head and brain.

Carotid endarterectomy. Surgical removal of deposits in the walls of the carotid artery that, when present, have the effect of narrowing its lumen.

Cerebrum. The main portion of the brain that includes the two cerebral hemispheres; this term is also used to refer to the entire brain.

Cognition/cognitive. The process of knowing, including awareness, perception, reasoning, remembering, and problem solving.

Contracture. A condition of fixed, high resistance to passive stretching that results from fibrosis and shortening of tissues that support muscles or joints.

Contralateral. The opposite side of the body.

Coronary heart disease. Deterioration of the heart caused by narrowing or clogging of arteries supplying the heart muscles, with resulting chest pain, heart attacks, and damage to the heart.

Decubitus ulcer. Ulcer of the skin that forms as a result of prolonged pressure in patients confined to bed or wheelchair.

Deep vein thrombosis (DVT). The clotting of blood in the deep veins of the leg or arm.

Dementia. A mental disorder characterized by the loss of intellectual abilities and, frequently, personality changes due to deterioration of the brain. Alzheimer's disease is a frequent example.

Depression. A mental state marked by feelings of despair, discouragement, and sadness.

Diagnosis. Determining the exact nature of a specific disease.

Dysarthria. A motor disorder that results in difficulty in motor speech mechanisms.

Dysphagia. Difficulty swallowing.

Embolus/embolism. A blood clot or other foreign substance that travels in the bloodstream to occlude an artery or vein.

Feeding gastrostomy. A surgical opening in the stomach through which a person is fed.

Graphesthesia. The sense by which figures or numbers drawn on the skin with a dull point are recognized.

Hemi-inattention. A disturbance of a person's awareness of space on the side of the body opposite a stroke-causing lesion; often referred to as unilateral neglect.

Hemiparesis. Muscular weakness or partial paralysis of one side of the body.

Hemiplegia. Paralysis of one side of the body.

Hemorrhage. Bleeding from the rupture of a blood vessel.

Hemorrhagic stroke. A stroke resulting from the rupture of a blood vessel in the brain.

Homonymous hemianopsia. Defective vision or blindness affecting the right or left halves of the visual fields of both eyes.

Hyperlipidemia. The state of having elevated lipid levels in the blood.

Hypertension. Elevated blood pressure.

Hypoarousal. Below normal level of arousal.

Incontinence. Lack of control over excretory functions (urination, bowels).

Infarction. Death of a part of an organ, such as the brain, due to lack of oxygen and other nutrients.

Ipsilateral. The same side of the body.

Intracerebral hemorrhage. Hemorrhage into the cerebrum.

Ischemic stroke. A stroke caused by an insufficient supply of blood and oxygen to a part of the brain.

Neurogenic bladder. Abnormal function of the urinary bladder due to damage to the nervous system.

Neurology. The branch of medicine that focuses on the study of the nervous system.

Occlusion. Blockage.

Orthostatic hypotension. Lowering of blood pressure with a change of body position from supine to erect.

Orthostatic tolerance. The ability to maintain blood pressure while standing upright.

Perception. Conscious mental recognition of a sensory stimulus.

Perseveration. Involuntary and pathologic persistence of the same verbal response or motor activity regardless of the stimulus or its duration.

Pressure ulcer. See decubitus ulcer.

Proprioception. Perception of body movement or position.

Spasticity. Abnormally increased tone in a muscle.

Stenosis. Reduction in the size of a vessel or other opening.

Stereognosis. The ability to perceive the nature and form of objects by the sense of touch.

Stroke. An acute neurological dysfunction of vascular origin with symptoms and signs corresponding to the involvement of focal areas of the brain; alternatively, the rapid onset of a neurological deficit that persists for at least 24 hours and is caused by intracerebral or subarachnoid hemorrhage or the blockage of a blood vessel supplying or draining the brain.

Subarachnoid hemorrhage. A hemorrhage in the space underneath the subarachnoid membrane that results in pressure on the brain or bleeding into the brain.

Thromboembolism. An embolus that originates in and breaks away from a clot in one vessel to become lodged in another vessel.

Thrombosis. The clotting of blood within a blood vessel.

Transient ischemic attack (TIA). The rapid onset of a neurological deficit that clears spontaneously in minutes or a few hours.

Unilateral neglect. A disturbance of a person's awareness of space on the side of the body opposite a stroke-causing lesion; often referred to as hemi-inattention.

Terms in Research Studies on Stroke Rehabilitation

Case fatality rate. The mortality rate in people affected with a given disease.

Control group. A group of subjects in a research study to which results of an experimental treatment given to another group of subjects are compared.

Epidemiology. The study of factors that influence the frequency and distribution of a disease in a population.

Experimental group. The group of subjects in a research study which receives the experimental treatment.

Experimental study. A study in which one treatment is compared to another.

Incidence. The frequency of occurrence of new cases of a disease over a specified period of time.

Meta-analysis. A technique for combining the results of several studies for the purpose of determining the net effects of related factors or treatments on a process or disease.

Multivariate analysis. A set of statistical techniques for analyzing the individual and joint effects of a number of factors on the outcomes of the process or disease being studied.

Observational study. A study that draws conclusions on the effects of factors or treatments by observing a group of subjects over a period of time.

Prospective study. A study that depends on data collected prospectively from the time the study begins.

Randomized controlled trial (RCT). A study in which subjects are assigned to the experimental or control group by a random selection procedure before data collection begins.

Retrospective study. A study that depends on data collected earlier, usually for purposes unrelated to the study.

Risk factor. A characteristic of the individual or environment that predisposes to the condition or disease of interest.

Contributors

Post-Stroke Rehabilitation Guideline Panel

Glen E. Gresham, MD, ***Chair***
Professor and Chairman
Department of Rehabilitation Medicine
State University of New York at Buffalo
Director of Rehabilitation Medicine
Erie County Medical Center
Buffalo, NY

Dr. Gresham is Professor and Chairman of Rehabilitation Medicine at the State University of New York at Buffalo. He was educated at Harvard College and Columbia University and received his clinical training in internal medicine at the University Hospitals of Cleveland. He has served on the faculties of Ohio State University, Yale University, Tufts University, and the State University at Buffalo.

Dr. Gresham became interested in stroke outcomes research in 1970. He published the first description of long-term disability outcomes in the Framingham Stroke Study, plus other analyses of stroke outcome. He continues as a consultant to the Framingham Stroke Study and has written extensive review articles, editorials, and chapters on stroke outcomes research. He is a member of the editorial board of *Stroke: A Journal of Cerebral Circulation.* In 1984, he and Carl V. Granger, MD, co-edited *Functional Assessment in Rehabilitation Medicine*, one of the first books in this field. In 1989, he organized an international symposium, "Methodologic Issues in Stroke Outcome Research," which was published as a supplement to *Stroke: A Journal of Cerebral Circulation.*

Dr. Gresham is a member of the Stroke Council of the American Heart Association and the American Congress of Rehabilitation Medicine. In 1992, he participated on the faculty of the Second World Congress of the International Stroke Society. He is the author of the chapter on stroke rehabilitation in both the first and second editions of *Stroke: Pathophysiology, Diagnosis, and Management*, edited by H.J.M. Barnett, J.P. Mohr, B.M. Stein, and F.M. Yatsu.

Pamela W. Duncan, PhD, PT, ***Co-Chair***
Associate Professor, Health Services Administration
University of Kansas
Director of Research, Center on Aging
Kansas University Medical Center
Kansas City, KS

Dr. Duncan received her BS in physical therapy from Columbia University and her PhD in epidemiology from the University of

North Carolina at Chapel Hill. During the preparation of this guideline, Dr. Duncan was an associate professor of physical therapy in the graduate program at Duke University. Also at Duke, she served as a research associate professor in the Center for Health Policy Research and Education, as well as a senior fellow in the Center for Aging and Human Development. From 1991 to 1994, she served as project director for the Stroke PORT, a 5-year study of secondary and tertiary prevention of stroke, funded by the Agency for Health Care Policy and Research. She is coinvestigator in Duke University's Claude Pepper Older American Independence Center Research.

Dr. Duncan is co-author of a book on stroke, *Stroke Rehabilitation: Recovery of Motor Control.* She has authored several papers on measurement and recovery of motor function following stroke. She has contributed to many publications on the measurement of physical performance in the frail elderly, and assessment of falls and imbalance in the elderly. Dr. Duncan has served the American Physical Therapy Association in many capacities and is immediate past president of the neurology section. She is a fellow of the Stroke Council of the American Heart Association and a member of the board of directors of the National Stroke Association.

In August 1994, she joined the faculty of the University of Kansas to develop a research program in geriatric rehabilitation outcomes and physical disability.

Harold P. Adams, Jr., MD
Professor of Neurology
Director, Division of Cerebrovascular Diseases
University of Iowa College of Medicine
Iowa City, IA

Dr. Adams is Professor and Director of the Division of Cerebrovascular Diseases, Department of Neurology, University of Iowa College of Medicine. His undergraduate education was at Drake University and the University of South Dakota. He received his MD degree from Northwestern University and performed his residency in neurology at the University of Iowa. He is certified in neurology by the American Board of Psychiatry and Neurology. Dr. Adams is a fellow of the American Academy of Neurology, American College of Physicians, and Stroke Council of the American Heart Association. He is also a member of the American Neurological Association. He serves on the editorial or advisory boards of *Stroke, Cerebrovascular Diseases,* and *Journal of Stroke and Cerebrovascular Disease.*

Dr. Adams has authored approximately 190 papers and chapters, largely dealing with stroke. He edited the *Handbook of Cerebrovascular Diseases*, which appeared in 1993. He has participated in a number of clinical studies and trials in stroke and is principal investigator of a

NINDS-funded randomized trial that is testing the usefulness of heparinoid, Org 10172, in improving outcome after stroke. The Stroke Council of the American Heart Association named Dr. Adams as recipient of the 1993 Humana Award for excellence in clinical stroke research.

Alan M. Adelman, MD, MS
Associate Professor and Director of Research
Department of Family and Community Medicine
Pennsylvania State University
The Milton S. Hershey Medical Center
Hershey, PA

Dr. Adelman is Associate Professor and Director of Research in the Department of Family and Community Medicine, Pennsylvania State University. He received his MD degree in 1975 from Temple University School of Medicine, Philadelphia, Pennsylvania. He performed his residency training in family medicine at Kaiser Foundation Hospital in Los Angeles, California. Upon completing his residency training, he served 3 years in the U.S. Public Health Service at the Keams Canyon Indian Health Service Hospital, Keams Canyon, Arizona.

He completed a Robert Woods Johnson Family Practice Faculty Development Fellowship at the University of Iowa in 1983. At that time, he also received a master's degree in preventive medicine. He has served on the faculties of the Department of Family Medicine at the University of Connecticut and University of Maryland, prior to his current position at the Hershey Medical Center. He has extensive experience and added qualifications in geriatrics. Prior to his present appointment, Dr. Adelman served as the medical director of the geriatric rehabilitation unit at the James Lawrence Kernan Hospital, Baltimore, Maryland (an affiliate of the University of Maryland Medical System).

David N. Alexander, MD
Director of Stroke Rehabilitation
Center for Diagnostic and Rehabilitation Medicine
Daniel Freeman Hospital
Assistant Clinical Professor, Department of Neurology
University of California at Los Angeles School of Medicine
Los Angeles, CA

Dr. Alexander is a neurologist whose primary clinical focus for the past 10 years has been on neurological rehabilitation. Currently, he is the Director of Stroke Rehabilitation at the Center for Diagnostic and Rehabilitation Medicine at Daniel Freeman Hospital, and Associate Clinical Professor at the UCLA School of Medicine, Department of Neurology. An honors graduate both of Amherst College and the University of Minnesota Medical School, Dr. Alexander was an intern in medicine at University Hospital in Boston and a resident in neurology at the Neurological Institute of New York at Columbia-Presbyterian Medical Center. He is actively engaged in clinical research, scholarly publication, and teaching of neurorehabilitation. He is a fellow of the Stroke Council of the American Heart Association, a site surveyor for the Commission on Accreditation of Rehabilitation Facilities, and a member of the American Society of Neurorehabilitation.

Duane S. Bishop, MD
Director, Rehabilitation Psychiatry
Rhode Island Hospital
Associate Professor, Department of Psychiatry
Brown University
Providence, RI

Dr. Bishop received his MD at the University of Alberta, Canada, and completed his residency in psychiatry at the McMaster University, Canada. Dr. Bishop is Associate Professor of Psychiatry, Department of Psychiatry and Human Behavior, Brown University, Providence, Rhode Island, and also the Director of Rehabilitation Psychiatry at Rhode Island Hospital in Providence. Along with Dr. Nathan Epstein, he was an originator of the McMaster Model of Family Functioning and the Problem Centered Systems Therapy of the Family Model, the McMaster Family Assessment Device (FAD), and the McMaster Clinical Rating Scale (CRS). He led the group's development of the McMaster Structured Interview of Family Functioning (McSIFF). Dr. Bishop has completed numerous research studies on the families of psychiatric and chronic illness (including stroke) populations. Dr. Bishop has published more than 90 articles and abstracts, has been a visiting professor at several international universities, and has made many national and international presentations.

Leonard Diller, PhD
Chief, Behavioral Science
Professor, Clinical Rehabilitation Medicine
Rusk Institute of Rehabilitation Medicine
New York University Medical Center
New York, NY

Dr. Diller received his PhD in clinical psychology from New York University in 1953. Since 1952, he has been associated with the Rusk Institute of Rehabilitation Medicine at NYU Medical Center. He is currently Chief of Psychological Services and Director of Behavioral Sciences. Dr. Diller has been a professor of clinical rehabilitation medicine since 1972.

His research has been in the development of approaches to improve cognitive deficits in individuals with brain damage. He has directed a number of federally funded research programs and is currently the director of a research and training center in head trauma and stroke, sponsored by the National Institute on Disability and Rehabilitation Research. He has authored more than 100 articles in the professional literature.

Dr. Diller has served as president of the American Congress of Rehabilitation Medicine and president of the Rehabilitation Psychological Association, and has been program committee chairman of the International Neuropsychological Society. He has been a grant reviewer for the major Federal research agencies; and he has been on the editorial boards of nine major journals in the field.

Dr. Diller was the first recipient of the Hayden Williams Fellowship of the Western Australian Institute of Technology in studies in psychology and the Caveness Memorial Award of the National Head Injury Foundation. He has received meritorious service awards from the New York State United Cerebral Palsy Association and the New York Chapter of the National Rehabilitation Association. In 1992, he was a recipient of the Gold Key Award from the American Congress of Rehabilitation Medicine.

Nancy E. Donaldson, RN, DNSc
Consumer Representative
Newport Beach, CA

Dr. Donaldson received her nursing degree and master's of nursing science from California State University at Los Angeles and her doctorate from the University of California at San Francisco. Dr. Donaldson (Mrs. Stephen E. Donaldson) has a longstanding interest in family adaptation during transitions in health. Following her husband's stroke in 1989, she experienced firsthand the demands and challenges of family adaptation and caregiving. Formerly, she served as the principal investigator, Orange County Research Utilization in Nursing Project. Dr. Donaldson is the Executive Director, Clinical Effectiveness, Quality Outcomes Management Services, UniHealth America, Burbank, California.

Carl V. Granger, MD
Professor of Rehabilitation Medicine
Director, Center for Functional Assessment Research
State University of New York at Buffalo
Buffalo, NY

Dr. Granger received his MD from New York University. Since 1983, he has been Professor of Rehabilitation Medicine at the State University of New York at Buffalo. He was also the former head of the Department of Rehabilitation Medicine at Buffalo General Hospital. He is Associate Chairman of Rehabilitation Medicine, Director of the Center for Functional Assessment Research, Department of Rehabilitation Medicine, and Co-Director of the University at Buffalo Multiple Sclerosis Center.

Dr. Granger has completed more than 80 publications, including "Outcome of Comprehensive Medical Rehabilitation: Measurement by

PULSES Profile and the Barthel Index," in collaboration with G.L. Albrecht and B.B. Hamilton. This journal article appeared in *Archives of Physical Medicine and Rehabilitation* (1979). He has been awarded the Elizabeth and Sidney Licht Award for Excellence in Scientific Writing. He is also co-editor with G.E. Gresham of *Functional Assessment in Rehabilitation Medicine* (Williams & Wilkins, 1984), and co-author with G.B. Seltzer and C. Fishbein of *Primary Care of the Functionally Disabled* (Lippincott, 1987).

Audrey L. Holland, PhD
Professor and Head
Department of Speech and Hearing Sciences
University of Arizona
Tucson, AZ

Audrey L. Holland received her PhD from the University of Pittsburgh. Currently, she is Professor and Head, Department of Speech and Hearing Sciences, University of Arizona. The major focus of her research, clinical service, and teaching has been on neurogenic communication disorders, with a primary emphasis on clinically relevant research in aphasia. She has served on the advisory board of the National Institute of Deafness and Other Communication Disorders, as well as on the editorial boards of a number of professional journals, and recently completed a term as chair of the board of governors of the Academy of Aphasia. She has published more than 100 articles related to neurogenic communication disorders, and frequently lectures on clinical management of aphasia and related problems. In 1990, she received the honors of the association from the American-Speech-Language-Hearing Association.

Margaret Kelly-Hayes, EdD, RN, CRRN
Research Coordinator and Investigator
Neuroepidemiology Section, Department of Neurology
Boston University School of Medicine
Boston, MA

Dr. Kelly-Hayes is Associate Clinical Professor of Neurology (neurological nursing) at Boston University School of Medicine and Neurology Projects Director, the Framingham Stroke Study. Her degrees include a BS in nursing from Boston College, a master's in rehabilitation nursing, and a doctorate in health education from Boston University. Dr. Kelly-Hayes' research activities focus on the neuroepidemiology of stroke. She has authored numerous articles on rehabilitation nursing, stroke prevention, and post-stroke recovery. In 1991, she was co-editor for *Nursing Clinics of North America* on stroke. Dr. Kelly-Hayes has represented rehabilitation nursing on several national committees, including the national advisory board for the Uniform Data System for Medical

Rehabilitation. She is also an elected fellow to the American Heart Association's Council on Stroke.

Fletcher H. McDowell, MD
Executive Medical Director, Burke Rehabilitation Hospital
White Plains, NY
Associate Dean and Winifred Masterson Burke Professor of Neurology and Rehabilitation Medicine
Cornell University Medical College
New York, NY

Dr. McDowell is the Winifred Masterson Burke Professor of Rehabilitation Medicine at Cornell University Medical College and is Professor of Neurology at Cornell University Medical College. He is currently the Executive Medical Director of the Burke Rehabilitation Hospital, White Plains, New York. He is also the Associate Dean of Cornell University Medical College.

Dr. McDowell is a graduate of Dartmouth College and received his MD from Cornell University Medical College in New York City. He has served as chairman of the board of directors of the National Stroke Association and is currently the president of the organization.

Dr. McDowell has published extensively on clinical neurology, stroke, Parkinson's disease, and rehabilitation medicine. He is past editor of the American Heart Association's journal *Stroke* and is currently an associate editor of the journal of *Stroke and Cerebral Vascular Disease*. He is a member of the American Neurological Association and the American Academy of Neurology.

Larry R. Myers, MD
Clinician, Office-Based Practice
Ambulatory Sentinel Practice Network
Community Preceptor
Mansfield, TX

Dr. Myers is a residency-trained family physician, practicing rural and semirural primary care for 15 years. Initially trained as a fighter pilot in Vietnam (following graduation from the Naval Academy at Annapolis), he received his medical education at the University of Arizona. Following residency training at the Medical University of South Carolina, he began practicing rural medicine as part of the Robert Wood Johnson Foundation's Rural Practice Project in northern Michigan. Subsequently, he has joined his practice in Texas, as a research clinician with the Ambulatory Sentinel Practice Network, an affiliation of primary care practices across the United States and Canada. (Dr. Myers also practices rural emergency medicine.)

He is a member of the American Academy of Family Physicians, Society of Teachers of Family Medicine, and NAPCRG. His primary interests are rural primary care, illness behavior, and geriatrics.

Marion A. Phipps, RN, MS, CRRN, FAAN
Rehabilitation Nurse Specialist
Beth Israel Hospital
Boston, MA

Marion Phipps is a rehabilitation nurse specialist at the Beth Israel Hospital in Boston, Massachusetts. Ms. Phipps received her nursing degree from the University of New Hampshire and a master's in rehabilitation nursing from Boston University. Her areas of interest include the application of rehabilitation nursing approaches in the acute care setting, care of stroke patients, and geriatric rehabilitation. Ms. Phipps is a fellow of the American Academy of Nursing and a member of Sigma Theta Tau. She is certified in rehabilitation nursing and is an active member of the Association of Rehabilitation Nurses (having served on local and national committees). Ms. Phipps has written numerous rehabilitation nursing articles, and she served as a guest editor for the 1991 Stroke Symposium in Nursing Clinics of North America.

Elliot J. Roth, MD
Director, Rehabilitation Institute of Chicago
Professor, Department of Physical Medicine and Rehabilitation
Northwestern University Medical School
Chicago, IL

Dr. Roth received his AB in chemistry and human services education from the Washington University, St. Louis. He received his MD from the Northwestern University Medical School. Dr. Roth interned at Cook County Hospital in Chicago, and he completed his residency and fellowship at the Northwestern University Medical School/Rehabilitation Institute of Chicago.

Dr. Roth is Director of the Rehabilitation Institute of Chicago and Professor of Physical Medicine and Rehabilitation at Northwestern University Medical School. He has also served as associate director of spinal cord injury rehabilitation for the Midwest Regional Spinal Cord Injury Care System.

He has published numerous peer-reviewed papers, reviews, and chapters on a variety of topics related to stroke and rehabilitation, and he has directed several research grants. Dr. Roth gives more than 50 lectures a year and recently received an outstanding teaching award. He serves on the editorial boards of several journals and is chairman of the rehabilitation committee of the American Heart Association of Metropolitan Chicago. Dr. Roth's clinical and academic interests are in the areas of comorbidity, outcome assessment, and rehabilitation management of stroke patients.

Hilary C. Siebens, MD
Medical Director, Skilled Nursing and Assessment Center
Medical Director, Rehabilitation Research
Cedars Sinai Medical Center
Assistant Clinical Professor
Department of Medicine, Division of Physical Medicine and Rehabilitation
University of California at Los Angeles
Los Angeles, CA

Dr. Siebens received her MD from Harvard Medical School, her board certification in internal medicine after training at Johns Hopkins Hospital, her special qualifications in geriatric medicine after a geriatric fellowship at Harvard University, and her board certification in physical medicine and rehabilitation after a residency at Tufts University.

She currently is Assistant Medical Director, Department of Physical Medicine and Rehabilitation, Cedar-Sinai Medical Center, Los Angeles, California. At UCLA, she is an assistant clinical professor in the Department of Medicine/Geriatric Medicine, Division of Physical Medicine and Rehabilitation. Her clinical work over the past 6 years has included treatment of 450 stroke inpatients, 1,200 rehabilitation outpatient visits, 1,300 acute hospital consultations, and medical directorship of the Cedar-Sinai Medical Center's 30-bed hospital-based skilled nursing facility.

Dr. Siebens has received research support from the Eleanor Naylor Dana Charitable Trust for a study on blood volumes after hip fracture, from NIH for a pilot study on stroke outcomes, and from the John A. Hartford Foundation for a randomized controlled trial of exercise in older hospitalized patients. She has consulted on a multicenter HCFA study at the University of Colorado on stroke and hip fracture rehabilitation outcomes. She has also consulted on a Robert Wood Johnson-funded study on innovative rehabilitation care outcomes in stroke, hip fracture, and medical/surgical patients.

She has published original research on eating disabilities, normal blood volumes in older adults, and blood volumes after vascular surgery and hip fracture; and review chapters on the topics of geriatric rehabilitation, medications in older rehabilitation patients, and deconditioning in older adults.

Gloria A. Tarvin, MSW, LSW
Chairperson of Allied Health/Nursing
Director of Social Work
Rehabilitation Institute of Chicago
Chicago, IL

Gloria Tarvin is Chairperson of Allied Health/Nursing and Director of Social Work, Rehabilitation Institute of Chicago. She is an instructor of clinical rehabilitation in the Department of Physical Medicine and Rehabilitation at Northwestern University Medical School. She earned her

AB degree from Brown University and her MSW degree from Atlanta University School of Social Work.

Ms. Tarvin is currently on the board of directors of the Society of Social Work Administrators in Health Care of the American Hospital Association. She is on the consulting editor's board of *Health and Social Work*. Her teaching experience includes topics related to rehabilitation and social work, both clinical and administrative.

Catherine A. Trombly, ScD, OTR/L, FAOTA
Professor of Occupational Therapy
Sargent College of Allied Health Professions
Boston University
Boston, MA

Catherine Trombly is a certified and licensed occupational therapist and fellow of the American Occupational Therapy Association. She received her basic professional training in occupational therapy at the University of New Hampshire and completed graduate study in occupational therapy at the University of Southern California (MA) and at Boston University (ScD). Her area of specialization is adult physical dysfunction. Her clinical experience, obtained at Highland View Hospital in Cleveland, includes rehabilitation of patients with neurological disorders, especially stroke and spinal cord injury. Currently, she is Professor of Occupational Therapy, Sargent College of Allied Health Professions, Boston University.

Dr. Trombly is a charter member of the American Occupational Therapy Foundation's Academy of Research. Her primary post-stroke research interest is the study of the mechanisms of motor impairment, and the effectiveness of therapy to remediate those impairments.

Catherine Trombly is the editor and major author of *Occupational Therapy for Physical Dysfunction*, published by Williams & Wilkins. It was the first textbook for therapists and students interested in the treatment of physical disabilities. The fourth edition is now in progress.

Other Contributors[1]

Consultants

Robert F. Berrian, MA, CTRS
Director of Recreational Therapy Services
Health South Rehabilitation Center
Mechanicsburg, PA
Specialty: Therapeutic Recreation

Richard W. Bohannon, EdD, PT, NCS
Professor, School of Allied Health
University of Connecticut
Storrs, CT
Therapist, Hartford Hospital
Hartford, CT
Specialty: Physical Therapy

James S. Liljestrand, MD, MPH
Medical Director, Braintree Hospital
President, National Association of Rehabilitation Facilities
Braintree, MA
Specialty: Internal Medicine

Fay W. Whitney, RN, PhD, FAAN
Assistant Professor, School of Nursing
University of Pennsylvania
Philadelphia, PA
Specialty: Rehabilitation Nursing

Peer Reviewers, *Guideline Technical Report*

Michael Alexander, MD
Director, Stroke Rehabilitation
Braintree Hospital
Braintree, MA
Associate Professor of Neurology
Boston University
Boston, MA

Stephen N. Berk, PhD
Director, Department of Psychology
Moss Rehabilitation Hospital
Philadelphia, PA

Murray E. Brandstater, MBBS, PhD
Professor and Chairman
Department of Physical Medicine and Rehabilitation
School of Medicine
Loma Linda University
Loma Linda, CA

Kathryn S. Bronstein, PhD, RN
Clinical Nurse Specialist
Cerebrovascular Neurosurgery
Northwestern Medical Facility/Foundation
Chicago, IL

Bruce M. Caplan, PhD
Chief Psychologist and Associate Professor
Thomas Jefferson University Hospital
Department of Rehabilitation Medicine
Philadelphia, PA

Catherine A. Clancy, PhD, CSW-ACP
Director, Social Service Department
St. Luke's Episcopal Hospital
Houston, TX

---

[1]Being listed in this section does not necessarily imply endorsement of the guideline products.

Catherine Coyle, CTRS, PhD
Associate Professor
Temple University
Philadelphia, PA

Mary Dombovy, MD
Assistant Professor of Neurology and Rehabilitation
University of Rochester, New York
Chair, Department of Physical Medicine and Rehabilitation
St. Mary's Hospital
Rochester, NY

Nancy Doolittle, PhD, RN
Research Nurse
Department of Physiological Nursing
University of California, San Francisco
San Francisco, CA

Ron L. Evans, ACSW
Clinical Assistant Professor
University of Washington School of Medicine
Department of Rehabilitation Medicine
Seattle, WA

Mary M. Evert, MBA, OTR, FAOTA
President
American Occupational Therapy Association
McLean, VA

Carol Frattali, PhD
Director, Health Services Division
American Speech-Language-Hearing Association
Rockville, MD

Marcus J. Fuhrer, PhD
Director
National Center for Medical Rehabilitation Research
National Institute of Child Health and Human Development
Rockville, MD

Kenda Fuller, PT, NCS
Lutheran Hospital
Wheat Ridge, CO

Gary Goldberg, MD
Associate Professor
Department of Physical Medicine and Rehabilitation
Temple University School of Medicine
Consultant, Stroke Center
Moss Rehabilitation Hospital
Philadelphia, PA

Wayne A. Gordon, PhD
Professor and Associate Director
Mt. Sinai School of Medicine
New York, NY

Mark V. Johnston, PhD
Director of Outcome Research
Kessler Institute for Rehabilitation
University of Medicine and Dentistry of New Jersey/ New Jersey Medical School
West Orange, NJ

Lyn Jongbloed, OTR, PhD
Associate Professor
School of Rehabilitation Sciences
University of British Columbia
Vancouver, BC, Canada

Richard B. Lazar, MD
Executive Vice President,
Medical Director
Schwab Rehabilitation Hospital
Departments of Neurology and
Physical Medicine and
Rehabilitation
Northwestern University
Medical School
Chicago, IL

Jeri A. Logemann, PhD
Professor and Chairman
Department of Communication
Sciences and Disorders
Northwestern University
Evanston, IL

James Malec, PhD, LP, ABPP
Neuropsychologist
Mayo Medical Center
Rochester, MN

Richard S. Materson, MD
National Rehabilitation Hospital
Washington, DC

John Melvin, MD
Vice President of Medical Affairs
Moss Rehabilitation Hospital
Chairman, Physical Medicine
and Rehabilitation
Albert Einstein Medical Center
Professor and Deputy Chairman,
Department of Physical Medicine
and Rehabilitation
Temple University
Philadelphia, PA

Christina M. Mumma,
PhD, RN, CRRN
Associate Professor and Chair
Graduate Nursing Program
University of Alaska
Anchorage, AK

Kenneth Ottenbacher, PhD, OTR
Professor and Associate Dean
School of Health-Related
Professions
State University of New York
at Buffalo
East Amherst, NY

Walter Panis, MD
Assistant Director of Neurology
Spaulding Rehabilitation Hospital
Boston, MA

Frances Pendergraft
Executive Director
of Counseling Services
Institute for Rehabilitation
and Research
Houston, TX

Judith M. Popovich,
DNSc, RN, CRRN
Assistant Professor
College of Nursing
University of Kentucky
Lexington, KY

Thomas R. Price, MD
Professor of Neurology,
Epidemiology, and
Preventive Medicine
University of Maryland Hospital
Baltimore, MD

Michael J. Reding, MD
Associate Professor of Neurology
Cornell University
Medical College at
Burke Rehabilitation Hospital
White Plains, NY

J. Scott Richards, PhD
Director of Psychology
Spain Rehabilitation Center
Birmingham, AL

Jay H. Rosenberg, MD
Chairman, Quality Standards Subcommittee
American Academy of Neurology
Clinical Associate Professor of Neurology
University of California at San Diego School of Medicine
Staff Neurologist
Southern California Permanente Medical Group
San Diego, CA

Shirley A. Sahrmann, PhD, PT
Associate Professor, Physical Therapy and Neurology
Washington University School of Medicine
St. Louis, MO

Margaret Stinemen, MD
Assistant Professor of Rehabilitation Medicine
University of Pennsylvania
Philadelphia, PA

J. Paul Thomas, PhD
Director, Medical Sciences Programs
National Institute on Disability and Rehabilitation Research
U.S. Department of Education
Washington, DC

James F. Toole, MD
Director, Stroke Research Center
Bowman Gray School of Medicine
Winston-Salem, NC

Karin Mueck Vecchione, MEd, CTRS
Administrator, Senior Network, Inc.
Oxon Hill, MD

Derick T. Wade, MD
Consultant in Neurological Disability
Rivermead Rehabilitation Centre
Oxford, United Kingdom

Robert T. Wertz, PhD
VA-Vanderbilt Professor
Hearing and Speech Sciences
Vanderbilt University School of Medicine
VA Medical Center
Nashville, TN

Jack Whisnant, MD
Chair, Department of Health Services Research
Professor of Neurology
Mayo Medical School
Rochester, MN

Anne M. Woodson, OTR
University of Texas Medical Branch at Galveston
Galveston, TX

Kathryn M. Yorkston, PhD
Professor of Rehabilitation Medicine
University of Washington
Seattle, WA

Mark A. Young, MD
Department of Rehabilitation Medicine
Johns Hopkins University School of Medicine
Baltimore, MD

Richard Zorowitz, MD
Assistant Professor, Department of Physical Medicine and Rehabilitation
University of Medicine and Dentistry/New Jersey Medical School
Newark, NJ
Clinical Chief, Stroke Services
Kessler Institute for Rehabilitation
West Orange, NJ

Peer Reviewers: *Clinical Practice Guideline, Quick Reference Guide for Clinicians, and the Patient and Family Guide*

Vivian Beyda, DrPH, Director
Barrier Free Design
and Communication
New York, NY
Eastern Paralyzed Veterans Association

Joseph Bleiberg, PhD
Director of Psychology
National Rehabilitation Hospital
Washington, DC
American Psychological Association

Laura Todd Brown, PA-C
American Academy of
Physician Assistants
Aledo, TX
American Academy of Physician Assistants

Louis R. Caplan, MD
Department of Neurology
New England Medical Center
Boston, MA
American Academy of Neurology

Pat Carter
Associate Administrator
Hebrew Home
of Greater Washington
Rockville, MD
American Association of Homes for the Aging

Randall Cebul, MD
Associate Professor of Medicine
and Epidemiology, Biostatistics
Case Western Reserve University
MetroHealth Medical Center
Cleveland, OH
Society of General Internal Medicine

Gregg R. Clifford, MD
Consultants in Internal Medicine,
Ltd.
Norfolk, VA
American College of Physicians

Steven Cohen-Cole, MD
Wesley Woods Geriatric Hospital
Atlanta, GA
American Psychiatric Association

Gregory Jay Darby, PA-C
Rehabilitation Medicine
Association
Gainesville, FL
American Academy of Physician Assistants

Susan Dean-Baar,
PhD, RN, CRRN
Wheeling, IL
American Nurses Association

Alicejean L. Dodson, RN, MN
Washington, D.C.
American Health Care Association

Wayne R. English, DO, FAOCRM
Sportsmedicine Rehabilitation
Center
Bedford, TX
American Osteopathic Association

Bruce M. Gans, MD
President and CEO
Rehabilitation Institute
of Michigan
Detroit, MI
American Hospital Association

Arthur M. Gershkoff, MD
Clinical Director
Moss Rehabilitation Stroke Center
Philadelphia, PA
Moss Rehabilitation Hospital

Mary Jo Gibson
Senior Analyst
Public Policy Institute
Washington, DC
American Association of Retired Persons

Gary Goldberg, MD
Philadelphia, PA
American Academy of Physical Medicine and Rehabilitation

Elizabeth Gresch, President
Dow Chemical Company
Midland, MI
American College of Occupational and Environmental Medicine

Michael Hagen, MD
Associate Professor and Interim Chair
University of Kentucky, Department of Family Practice
Lexington, KY
American Academy of Family Physicians

Carolyn J. Harris, RN, BSN, MEd, NHA
Marlin Management Services, Inc.
Burlington, VT
American Health Care Association

Melinda Harrison
Director, Watson Clinic, Center for Rehabilitative Medicine
Lakeland, FL
American Speech-Language-Hearing Association

Jim Hinojosa, PhD, OTR, FAOTA
Associate Professor, Director of Post-Professional Graduate Program
Department of Occupational Therapy, New York University
New York, NY
American Occupational Therapy Association

Gary R. Houser
President, National Stroke Association
Englewood, CO
National Stroke Association

Jeanette Hoyt, CRRN
Willamette Falls Hospital–Home Health Agency
Oregon City, OR
National Association for Home Care

Katherine F. Jeter, EdD, ET
Executive Director
Help for Incontinent People, Inc.
Spartanburg, SC
Help for Incontinent People, Inc.

Philip W. Kassirer, PT
Director of Therapeutic Services
HCR–Home Health Agency
Rochester, NY
National Association for Home Care

Kathleen Kelly
Executive Director
Family Caregiver Alliance
San Francisco, CA
Family Caregiver Alliance

Evelyn Kennedy
Executive Director
Promote Real Independence for the Disabled and Elderly
Groton, CT
Promote Real Independence for the Disabled and Elderly

Corinne Kirchner, PhD
Director of Social Research
American Foundation for the Blind
New York, NY
American Foundation for the Blind

Paul Leung, PhD
Division of Rehabilitation Education Services
University of Illinois
Champaign, IL
American Psychological Association

Sharon M. Lyke, RN, BSN, CRRN
Hilltop Home Care
Grand Junction, CO
National Association for Home Care

Marjorie A. Maddox, ARNP, ANP-C
University of Louisville, School of Nursing
Louisville, KY
American Academy of Nurse Practitioners

Jane Mathews-Gentry, PT, MPH, DSc
Rehabilitation Supervisor
VNA/North Shore, Inc.
Danvers, MA
National Association for Home Care

John L. Melvin, MD
Philadelphia, PA
National Association of Rehabilitation Facilities

Stephanie Mensh
Falls Church, VA
American Urological Association

John Murphy, MD
Washington, DC
Gerontological Society of America

Jonathan Musher, MD
Vice President of Medical Affairs
Beverly Enterprises
Fort Smith, AR
American Health Care Association

Glenn E. Nancarrow, PT
Santa Fe Home Care
Gainesville, FL
National Association for Home Care

Jane M. O'Toole, ARNP
Santa Fe Home Care
Gainesville, FL
National Association for Home Care

Alberta Orr, MSW
National Program Associate
American Foundation for the Blind
New York, NY
American Foundation for the Blind

Robin J. Patterson, BSN, RN
Quality Validation Specialist
Unicare Health Facilities, Inc.
Spokane, WA
American Health Care Association

Kriste Petite, RN, MSN, COHN
Intel Corporation
Santa Clara, CA
American Association of Occupational Health Nurses

Marcia B. Richards, RN, RS
Washington, DC
American Health Care Association

Robert Robinson, MD
Department of Psychiatry
University of Iowa Hospitals and Clinics
Iowa City, IA
American Psychiatric Association

H. Denman Scott, MD, FACP
Philadelphia, PA
American College of Physicians

Thomas K. Skalko, PhD, CTRS
Florida International University
Miami, FL
American Therapeutic Recreation Association

Andrew H. Smith
Research Analyst
American Association of Retired Persons
Washington, DC
American Association of Retired Persons

Mary T. St. Pierre
Associate Director of Regulatory Affairs
National Association for Home Care
Washington, DC
National Association for Home Care

Joan Unger, RN/ARNP-C, MS, CNA
Land o' Lakes, FL
American Academy of Nurse Practitioners

Donna L. Wagner, PhD
Vice President of Programs
National Council on the Aging, Inc.
Washington, DC
National Council on the Aging, Inc.

Sandra M. Watchous, MN, RN
Hays, KS
National Association for Home Care

Barb Wegener, RN, BSN, MPA, CNAA
Program Manager: Specialty Services
Brevard Home Care
Wuestoff Health Systems
Melbourne, FL
National Association for Home Care

Leon A. Weisberg, MD
Tulane University School of Medicine
Department of Psychiatry and Neurology
New Orleans, LA
American Society of Internal Medicine

Rita Wray, BSN, CNA
Brandon, MS
National Black Nurses Association

Kathleen Wreford, RD
American Dietetic Association
Clinical Dietitian
Rehabilitation Institute of Michigan
Detroit, MI
American Dietetic Association

Site Testers

Helen S. Philliou, RN, BS
Case Management Consultant
Winchester, MA

LaDonna Reading
Director of Clinical Services
Continental Medical Systems
Mechanicsburg, PA

Joseph W. Vick Roy, MD
HEALTHSOUTH
Rehabilitation Hospital of Utah
Sandy, UT

Joanne Buttery, MSc
Stroke Team Coordinator
Timothy Meagher, MD
Christiane Gauthier, PhT
Physiotherapy
Lawrence Green, MD
Lilian Heimbach, OT, BSc
Occupational Therapy
Diane Larochelle, BSW
Louisette LaRochelle, BSW
Social Work
Annick Leboeuf-Lorange, BSc
Nursing
Judith Robillard Shultz, MSc
Speech-Language Pathology
Montreal General Hospital
Montreal, Quebec, Canada

John B. Anderson, MD, FRCP
Department of Neurology
Permanente Medical Group, Inc.
Oakland, CA

G. Nancy McGowan, RN, BSN, CRRN
Director of Utilization Management
Olsten Kimberly Quality Care
Westbury, NY

John A. Schuchmann, MD
Chairman
Scott and White Clinic
Temple, TX

Mary Finn, OTR/L
Coordinator of Program Evaluation
Spaulding Rehabilitation Hospital
Boston, MA

Catherine Kroll, DO
Gwinn Medical Center
UPRNet
Gwinn, MI

Marcie Barnette, RN, MSN, FNP
Director of Clinical Services
VNA of Washington, DC

Keith Rafal, MD
Regional Medical Director
Susan Anderson, MS, CCC
Speech-Language Pathologist
Mindy Grodofsky-Gilmore, LICSW, BCD
Nancy A. Lowenstein, MS, OTR
Jeanne Stack, RN
Senior Resource Clinician
Wellmark Health Care Services
Wellesley, MA

Organizations and Individuals Providing Additional Scientific, Technical, and Administrative Support

Center for Health Economics Research

William B. Stason, MD, MS
Project Director

A. James Lee, PhD
Project Manager/Economist

Ann Venable, MA
Scientific Writer

Cheryl S. Lewis
Administrative Assistant

Carol J. Ammering
Analyst

Monika Reti
Analyst

Holly A. Cyr
Analyst

Joyce Huber, PhD
Senior Economist

Helen Margulis, MS
Programmer

Robyn Tarantino
Programmer

Philip W. Tyo
Administrative Assistant

Adam J. Falk
Analyst

Amy Rensko
Analyst

Harvard School of Public Health

Sidney Klawansky, MD, PhD
Thomas Chalmers, MD
Meta-Analysis

Massachusetts PRO

Peter Maselli, MD
Medical Director
Review Criteria

Agency for Health Care Policy and Research

Douglas B. Kamerow, MD, MPH
Director, Office of the Forum for Quality and Effectiveness in Health Care

David C. Lanier, MD
Project Officer

Timothy F. Campbell
Managing Editor

Valna Montgomery
Product Manager

Attachments

Recommended standardized assessment instruments for use with stroke patients

1. Level-of-consciousness scale
2. Stroke deficit scales
3. Global disability scale
4. Measures of disability in basic activities of daily living (ADL)
5. Mental status screening tests
6. Assessment of motor function
7. Balance assessment
8. Mobility assessment
9. Assessment of speech and language functions
10. Depression scales
11. Measures of instrumental activities of daily living (IADL)
12. Family assessment
13. Quality-of-life measures

The attachments consist of summary tables describing the preferred instruments. Clinicians desiring to use them with patients should use the referenced sources and obtain the actual assessments and accompanying instructions for administering and scoring purposes.

Attachment 1. Level-of-consciousness scale

Instrument	Description	Validity, reliability, and sensitivity	Uses and time to administer	Strengths and weaknesses
Glasgow Coma Scale[a,b]	3 sections scoring eye opening, motor, and verbal responses to voice commands or pain. Each section scored separately on scales ranging from 4 to 6 points.	Validity: Face and predictive validity well demonstrated.[b,c,**] Reliability: Interobserver reliability good.[d,**] Sensitivity: Reasonable.[b,*]	Use: Acute post-stroke period. Time: 2 minutes.	Strengths: Simple, valid, reliable, and widely used.

[a]Teasdale and Jennett, 1974.
[b]Teasdale, Murray, Parker, et al., 1979.
[c]Levy, Bates, Caroona, et al., 1981.
[d]Teasdale, Knill-Jones, and Van der Sande, 1978.

Note: * = adequately evaluated. ** = comprehensively evaluated.

Attachment 2. Stroke deficit scales

Instrument	Description	Validity, reliability, and sensitivity	Uses and time to administer	Strengths and weaknesses
NIH Stroke Scale[a]	15 items scored on 3- or 4-point interval scales. Domains: Consciousness, vision, extraocular movements, facial palsy, limb strength, ataxia, sensation, speech and language.	Validity: Good correlation with infarct volume and 3-month outcomes.[a,c,**] Reliability: Moderate interrater and intrarater reliability.[a,b,c,*]	Uses: Acute care screening, formal assessment, monitoring. Time: 5-10 minutes.	Strengths: Brief. Good reliability. Can be administered by nonneurologists. Weaknesses: Interval scale is relatively insensitive to change.
Canadian Neurological Scale[d]	8 items scored on a 3-point interval scale. Score is 10 in normal patients. Separate section measures face and motor responses in cognitively impaired patients. Domains: Consciousness, orientation, speech, motor function, facial weakness.	Validity: Established versus neurological examination and Katz ADL scores.[e,*] Reliability: Moderate interrater and intrarater reliability.[e,*]	Uses: Acute care, screening, formal assessment, monitoring. Time: 5 minutes.	Strengths: Brief. Valid with good reliability. Weaknesses: Omits ataxia, visual fields, eye movements. Interval scale relatively insensitive to change.

[a]Brott, Adams, Olinger, et al., 1989.
[b]Goldstein, Bertels, and Davis, 1989.
[c]Wityk, Pessin, Kaplan, et al., 1994.
[d]Cote, Hachinski, Shurvell, et al., 1986.
[e]Cote, Battista, Wolfson, et al., 1989.

Note: * = adequately evaluated. ** = comprehensively evaluated. ADL = activities of daily living.

Attachment 3. Global disability scale

Instrument	Description	Validity, reliability, and sensitivity	Uses and time to administer	Strengths and weaknesses
Rankin Scale[a] Scale Modification[b,c]	Ordinal scale with six grades indicating degrees of disability.	Validity[b,**] Reliability[c,*] Sensitivity: Not tested.	Uses: Acute hospitalization. Time: 5 minutes.	Strengths: Simple overall assessment of disability. Weaknesses: Walking the only explicit function assessed. Probably insensitive to change.

[a]Rankin, 1957.
[b]Bonita and Beaglehole, 1988.
[c]van Swieten, Koudstaal, Visser, et al., 1988.

Note: * = adequately evaluated. ** = comprehensively evaluated.

Attachment 4. Measures of disability in basic activities of daily living (ADL)

Instrument	Description	Validity, reliability, and sensitivity	Uses and time to administer	Strengths and weaknesses
Barthel Index[a,b]	Ordinal scale with total scores from 0 (totally dependent) to 20 (totally independent) (or, 0 to 100 by multiplying each item score by 5). 10 items: bowels, bladder, feeding, grooming, dressing, transfer, toilet use, mobility, stairs, bathing.	Validity[c,d,e,f,**] Reliability[b,g,**] Sensitivity[c,f,h,i,j,**]	Uses: Screening, formal assessment, monitoring, maintenance. Time: 5-10 minutes.	Strengths: Widely used in stroke disability. Excellent reliability and validity. Weaknesses: "Ceiling" effect in detecting change at higher level functioning. Only fair sensitivity to change.
Functional Independence Measure (FIM)[k,l,m,n]	18 items scored on a 7-point ordinal scale (1 = complete independence; 7 = total assistance). Total score ranges from 18 to 126. Subscores for motor function and cognition. Domains for self-care, sphincter control, mobility, locomotion, communication, and social cognition.	Validity[o,p,**] Reliability[o,q,**] Sensitivity[o,r,**]	Uses: Screening, formal assessment, monitoring, maintenance. Time: < 40 minutes.	Strengths: Measures social cognition and functional communication as well as mobility and ADL. Use of 7-point scale increases sensitivity versus other disability scales. Widely used in the United States and other countries. Weaknesses: "Ceiling" and "floor" effects at the upper and lower ends of function.

[a]Mahoney and Barthel, 1965.
[b]Wade and Collin, 1988.
[c]Gresham, Phillips, and Labi, 1980.
[d]Wade and Hewer, 1987a.
[e]Hertanu, Demopoulos, Yang, et al., 1984.
[f]Duncan, 1992.
[g]Shinar, Gross, Bronstein, et al., 1987.
[h]Shah, Vanclay, and Cooper, 1989.
[i]Granger, Albrecht, and Hamilton, 1979.
[j]Granger, Dewis, Peters, et al., 1979.
[k]Guide for the uniform data set for medical rehabilitation, 1993.
[l]Granger, Hamilton, Keith, et al., 1986.
[m]Granger, Hamilton, and Sherwin, 1986.
[n]Keith, Granger, Hamilton, et al., 1987.
[o]Hamilton, Granger, Sherwin, et al., 1987.
[p]Granger and Hamilton, 1990.
[q]Hamilton, Laughlin, Granger, et al., 1991.
[r]Granger and Hamilton, 1992.

Note: * = adequately evaluated. ** = comprehensively evaluated. ADL = activities of daily living. Additional useful instruments include the Katz Index of ADL (Katz, Ford, Moskowitz, et al., 1963), the Kenny Self-Care Evaluation (Schoening and Iversen,1968), LORS/LAD (Carey and Posavac,1978), and PECS (Harvey and Jellinek, 1981).

Attachment 5. Mental status screening tests

Instrument	Description	Validity, reliability, and sensitivity	Uses and time to administer	Strengths and weaknesses
Mini-Mental State Examination (MMSE)[a]	7 domains including orientation to time and place, registration of words, attention, calculation, recall, language, and visual construction.	Validity[a,b,*] Reliability[a,b,*] Sensitivity[b,c,d,*]	Uses: Screening. Time: < 10 minutes.	Strengths: Widely used for screening. Sensitive. Weaknesses: Several functions with summed score. May misclassify patients with aphasia. Education and normal aging must be considered in interpreting overall score.
Neurobehavioral Cognitive Status Examination (NCSE)[e,f]	10 scales: Graded assessment of function. Domains: Orientation, attention, comprehension, naming, construction, memory, calculation, similarities, judgment, and repetition.	Validity[f,g,h,i,*] Reliability: Not tested in stroke patients. Sensitivity[i,*]	Uses: Screening. Time: < 30 minutes.	Strengths: Predicts gain in Barthel Index score. Unrelated to age. Weaknesses: Does not distinguish right from left hemisphere strokes. No reliability studies on stroke. No studies of factorial structure. Correlates with education.[h]

[a]Folstein, Folstein, and McHugh, 1975.
[b]Tombaugh and McIntyre, 1992.
[c]Bachman, Wolf, Linn, et al., 1993.
[d]Tatemichi, Desmond, and Paik, 1991.
[e]Kiernan, 1987.
[f]Kiernan, Mueller, Langston, et al., 1987.
[g]Schwamm, Van Dyke, Keirnana, et al., 1987.
[h]Mysiw, Beegan, and Gatens, 1989.
[i]Osmon, Smet, Winegarden, et al., 1992.

Note: * = adequately evaluated. Another instrument, Motor Impersistence (Ben-Yishay, Diller, Gerstman, et al., 1968) focuses specifically on motor impersistence.

Attachment 6. Assessment of motor function

Instrument	Description	Validity, reliability, and sensitivity	Uses and time to administer	Strengths and weaknesses
Fugl-Meyer[a]	Measures impairment on a 3-point ordinal scale. Measurement of volitional movement is hierarchical. Sums are treated as continuous variables. Domains: Pain, range of motion, sensation, volitional movement, and balance.	Validity[a,b,c,d,e,**] Reliability[f,*] Sensitivity: Not formally tested but detected changes in cohorts of patients.[g]	Uses: Formal assessment, monitoring. Time: 30–40 minutes.	Strengths: Extensively evaluated measure. Good validity and reliability for assessing motor function and balance. Weaknesses: Many clinicians view the measure as too complex and time-consuming.
Motor Assessment Scale[h]	Measures impairment and disability on 6-point ordinal scale. Domains: Volitional arm and hand movements, tone, mobility (i.e., rolling, supine to sit, sitting, standing, walking).	Validity[i,*] Reliability[h,j,*] Sensitivity: Not tested.	Uses: Formal assessment, monitoring. Time: 15 minutes.	Strengths: Good reliability and validity. Weaknesses: Long to administer. Reliability assessed only in stable patients. Sensitivity to detect change not tested.
Motricity Index[k,l]	Measures impairment on a weighted ordinal scale. Domains: Strength and trunk control.	Validity[k,l,m,*] Reliability[l,*] Sensitivity: Not tested.	Uses: Screening, formal assessment, monitoring. Time: < 5 minutes.	Strengths: Brief assessment of motor function of arm, leg, and trunk. Weaknesses: Sensitivity to detect change not tested.

[a]Fugl-Meyer, Jaasko, Leyman, et al., 1975.
[b]Berglund and Fugl-Meyer, 1986.
[c]De Weerdt and Harrison, 1985.
[d]Wood-Dauphinee, Williams, and Shapiro, 1990.
[e]Dettmann, Linder, and Sepic, 1987.
[f]Duncan, Propst, and Nelson, 1983.
[g]Duncan, 1992.
[h]Carr, Shepherd, Nordholm, et al., 1985.
[i]Poole and Whitney, 1988.
[j]Loewen and Anderson, 1988.
[k]Demeurisse, Demol, and Robaye, 1980.
[l]Collin and Wade, 1990.
[m]Wade and Hewer, 1987a.

Note: * = adequately evaluated. ** = comprehensively evaluated.

Attachment 7. Balance assessment

Instrument	Description	Validity, reliability, and sensitivity	Uses and time to administer	Strengths and weaknesses
Berg Balance Scale[a,b]	Measures disability on 0–4 point ordinal scale. Domains: 14 items of balance.	Validity[a,b,**] Reliability[b,**] Sensitivity[b,*]	Uses: Formal assessment, monitoring. Time: < 10 minutes.	Strengths: Very simple measure of balance. Well characterized in stroke patients. Sensitive to change.

[a]Berg, Maki, Williams, et al., 1992.
[b]Berg, Wood-Dauphinee, Williams, et al., 1989.

Note: * = adequately evaluated. ** = comprehensively evaluated.

Attachment 8. Mobility assessment

Instrument	Description	Validity, reliability, and sensitivity	Uses and time to administer	Strengths and weaknesses
Rivermead Mobility Index[a,b]	Measures disability on a pass/fail scale. Domains: Turning over in bed, sitting, standing, transferring, and walking.	Validity[a,*] Reliability[a,*] Sensitivity[b,*]	Uses: Screening, formal assessment, monitoring. Time: < 5 minutes.	Strengths: Brief test of physical mobility. Reliable and valid.

[a]Wade, Collen, Robb, et al., 1992.
[b]Collen, Wade, Robb, et al., 1991.

Note: * = adequately evaluated.

Attachment 9. Assessment of speech and language functions

Instrument	Description	Validity, reliability, and sensitivity	Uses and time to administer	Strengths and weaknesses
Boston Diagnostic Aphasia Examination[a,b]	Assesses sample speech and language behavior on a 6-point ordinal scale. Modalities assessed: Fluency, naming, word finding, repetition, serial speech, auditory comprehension, reading, writing. Examiner judges grammar, syntax, frequency of paraphasias, and articulation.	Validity[b,*] Reliability: Not tested. Sensitivity: Not tested.	Uses: Formal assessment, monitoring. Time: 1-4 hours.	Strengths: Widely used, comprehensive, good standardization data, sound theoretical rationale. Weaknesses: Administration time long; half of patients cannot be classified.
Porch Index of Communicative Ability (PICA)[c]	Scored by a 16-point multidimensional scale with mean scores for entire test and each modality. Modalities assessed: Auditory comprehension, visual comprehension, written expression, verbal expression, and pantomime.	Validity: Standardized in 357 left, 96 right, and 100 bilateral hemisphere damaged subjects.[c,*] Reliability[c,*] Sensitivity: Not tested.	Uses: Formal assessment and monitoring. Time: 1/2-2 hours.	Strengths: Widely used, comprehensive, careful test development and standardization. Weaknesses: Requires special training to administer. Inadequate sampling of language other than one word and single sentences.
Western Aphasia Battery[d]	"Aphasia Quotient" and "Cortical Quotient." Scored on 100-point scale for both quotients. Modalities assessed: Spontaneous speech, repetition, comprehension, naming, reading, writing, construction, and Raven's Colored Progressive Matrices.	Validity: Standardized in 365 aphasic and 162 normal individuals. Correlations tested between 1977 and 1982 versions.[d,*] Reliability[d,*] Sensitivity: Not tested.	Uses: Formal assessment, monitoring. Time: 1-4 hours.	Strengths: Widely used, comprehensive. Weaknesses: Administration time long. "Aphasia quotient" and "taxonomy" of aphasia not well validated.

[a]Goodglass and Kaplan, 1972.
[b]Goodglass and Kaplan, 1983.
[c]Porch, 1981.
[d]Kertesz, 1982.

Note: * = adequately evaluated.

Attachment 10. Depression scales

Instrument	Description	Validity, reliability, and sensitivity	Uses and time to administer	Strengths and weaknesses
Beck Depression Inventory (BDI)[a,b]	Self-rating scale. 21 items (or 13 items in short form) with attitudinal, somatic, and behavioral components.	Validity: Concurrent validity versus the MMPI, Zung, Hamilton Rating Scale, and psychiatric ratings.** Reliability[a,c,d,*] Sensitivity[c,d,*]	Uses: Screening and monitoring. Time: 10 minutes.	Strengths: Widely used. Easily administered. Norms available. Good with somatic symptoms. Weaknesses: Less useful in elderly. Somatic items may not be due to depression. Aphasic patients have difficulty. Neglect patients cannot read items. High false positive rates. Face validity makes dissimulation easy.[e]
Center for Epidemiologic Studies Depression (CES-D)[f]	Self-rating scale that measures severity of depressive symptomatology. 20-item questionnaire investigating perceived mood and level of functioning within the past week.	Validity[f,g,h,*] Reliability[g,h,i,*] Sensitivity[g,*]	Uses: Screening and monitoring. Time: < 15 minutes.	Strengths: Brief self-report, easily administered. Useful in elderly. Effective for screening in stroke population. Weaknesses: Not appropriate for aphasic patients.
Geriatric Depression Scale (GDS)[j]	Self-rating scale with 30 items in yes/no format. No items refer to disability.	Validity: Concurrent versus Zung and Beck scales and Hamilton scale.[k,l,*] Reliability[k,*] Sensitivity[m,*]	Uses: Screening and monitoring. Time: 10 minutes.	Strengths: Brief. Less affected by visual impairments, physical illness, difficulty in choosing options, and poor motivation. Yes/no format better for elderly and cognitively impaired. Weaknesses: High false negative rates in minor depression.
Hamilton Depression Scale[n,o]	17-item observer-rated scale of somatic and nonsomatic symptoms.	Validity: Concurrent validity versus the present State Exam and Zung Depression Scale.[p,q,r,s,**] Reliability[r,s,t,u*]	Uses: Screening and monitoring. Time: < 30 minutes.	Strengths: Observer rated rather than self-report; frequently used in stroke patients; combined with Beck increases congruence with DSM-III-R criteria. Weaknesses: Multiple versions with different numbers of items and phrasing of questions compromise interobserver reliability.

Attachment 10. Depression scales (continued)

[a]Beck, Ward, Mendelson, et al., 1961.
[b]Beck and Steer, 1987.
[c]Schubert, Burns, Paras, et al., 1992a.
[d]Schubert, Burns, Paras, et al., 1992b.
[e]House, Dennis, Hawton, et al., 1989.
[f]Radloff, 1977.
[g]Shinar, Gross, Price, et al., 1986.
[h]Weissman, Sholomskas, Pottengel, et al., 1977.
[i]Parikh, Eden, Price, et al., 1988.
[j]Yesavage, Brink, Rose, et al., 1982-83.
[k]Norris, Gallager, Wilson, et al., 1987.
[l]Robinson and Price, 1982.
[m]Lichtenberg, Christensen, and Metler, 1993.
[n]Hamilton, 1960.
[o]Hamilton, 1967.
[p]Robinson, Parikh, Lipsey, et al., 1993.
[q]Robinson, Starr, Kubos, et al., 1983.
[r]Robinson, Starr, Lipsey, et al., 1985.
[s]Gordon, Hibbard, Egelko, et al., 1991.
[t]Williams, 1988.
[u]Robinson, Starr, Kubos, et al., 1983.

Note: * = adequately evaluated. ** = comprehensively evaluated. An additional well-validated instrument is the Zung Scale (Zung, 1965).

Attachment 11. Measures of instrumental activities of daily living (IADL)

Instrument	Description	Validity, reliability, and sensitivity	Uses and time to administer	Strengths and weaknesses
PGC Instrumental Activities of Daily Living[a]	Guttman scale with questions on use of telephone, walking, shopping, food preparation, housekeeping, laundry, public transportation, and medicine.	Validity[b,*] Reliability[a,c,d,*]	Uses: Maintenance. Time: < 30 minutes.	Strengths: Measures broad base of information necessary for independent living. Weaknesses: Has not been used in stroke population.
Frenchay Activities Index[e]	15 items concerning activities in and outside the home. Summary score (range 15-60 points) and subscale scores for domestic, leisure/work, and outdoor activities. Depends on patient and family self-reports.	Validity: Good correlation with Barthel Index and Sickness Impact Profile scores.[f,*]	Uses: Maintenance. Time: 10-15 minutes.	Strengths: Developed specifically for stroke patients. Assesses broad array of activities of daily living. Weaknesses: Sensitivity not tested but probably limited. Interobserver reliability not tested.

[a]Lawton, 1972.
[b]Rubenstein, Schairer, Wieland, et al., 1984.
[c]Lawton, 1988a.
[d]Lawton, 1988b.
[e]Holbrook and Skilbeck, 1983.
[f]Schuling, de Haan, Limburg, et al., 1993.

Note: * = adequately evaluated. Additional useful instruments include OARS: Instrumental ADL (Duke University, 1978), and the Functional Health Status (Rosow and Breslau, 1966).

Attachment 12. Family assessment

Instrument	Description	Validity, reliability, and sensitivity	Uses and time to administer	Strengths and weaknesses
Family Assessment Device (FAD)[a]	7 domain scales assessing problem solving, communication, roles, affective responsiveness, affective involvement, behavior control, and general functioning.	Validity[b,c,d,e,f,*] Reliability[a,c,e,g,*] Sensitivity: Not tested.	Uses: Formal assessment, monitoring, and maintenance. Time: < 30 minutes.	Strengths: Widely used in stroke. Computer scoring available. Excellent validity and reliability. Cut-off scores for family functioning. Available in multiple languages. Weaknesses: Assessment subjective. Sensitivity not tested.

[a]Epstein, Baldwin, and Bishop, 1983.
[b]Wenniger, Hagemand, and Arrindell, 1993.
[c]Byles, Bryne, Boyle, et al., 1988.
[d]Fristad, 1989.
[e]Miller, Bishop, Epstein, et al., 1985.
[f]Kabacoff, Miller, Bishop, et al., 1990.
[g]Kaufman, Tarnowski, Simonian, et al., 1991.

Note: * = adequately evaluated.

Attachment 13. Quality-of-life measures

Instrument	Description	Validity, reliability, and sensitivity	Uses and time to administer	Strengths and weaknesses
Medical Outcomes Study (MOS) 36-Item Short-Form Health Survey[a]	36 items with 118 levels. Domains: Physical functioning, role limitations due to physical or emotional problems, social functioning, bodily pain, mental health, vitality, and general health perceptions.	Validity: Well demonstrated for a derived 20-item scale.[a,**] Reliability: Well demonstrated for a derived 20-item scale.[a,**] Sensitivity: As sensitive as the Sickness Impact Profile.[b,*]	Uses: Maintenance. Time: 10-15 minutes.	Strengths: Improved version of SF-20. Eight scales are scored separately. All items are well standardized. Brief and can be self-completed or completed by telephone or personal interview. Widely used in the United States. Weaknesses: Possible "floor" effect in seriously ill patients, especially for physical functioning, suggests it should be supplemented by an ADL scale. Further validation studies in progress. Not tested in post-stroke rehabilitation patients.
Sickness Impact Profile (SIP)[c]	136 items with scores on subscales and summated. 12 subscales: Ambulation, mobility, body care, emotion, communication, alertness, sleep, eating, home management, recreation, social interactions, and employment.	Validity and reliability: Well demonstrated.[c,**] Sensitivity: Ability to detect change questioned.[d,*]	Uses: Maintenance. Time: 20-30 minutes.	Strengths: Comprehensive and well evaluated. Broad range of items reduces "floor" or "ceiling" effects. Weaknesses: Relatively long. Evaluates behavior rather than subjective health. Questions on well-being, happiness, and satisfaction should be added.

[a]Ware and Sherbourne, 1992.
[b]McHorney, Ware, Rogers, et al., 1992.
[c]Bergner, Bobbitt, Carter, et al., 1981.
[d]MacKenzie, Charlson, Digioia, et al., 1986.

Note: * = adequately evaluated. ** = comprehensively evaluated.

Index

D

E

F

G

H

I

J

L

M

N

O

P

T

U

V

W